Working as a
Nurse

Working as a
Nurse

*How to make your career
in a fulfilling profession*

**ESTHER BARTLETT
and
MARION FIELD**

How To Books

Published by How To Books Ltd.,
3 Newtec Place, Magdalen Road,
Oxford OX4 1RE, United Kingdom
Tel: 01865 793806   Fax: 01865 248780
email: info@howtobooks.co.uk
http://www.howtobooks.co.uk

British Library Cataloguing-in-Publication Data.
A catalogue record for this book is available from
the British Library.

Edited by Alison Wilson
Cover design by Shireen Nathoo Design
Cover image PhotoDisc

Produced for How To Books by Deer Park Productions
Typeset by Euroset, Alresford, Hampshire SO24 9PQ
Printed and bound by Cromwell Press, Trowbridge, Wiltshire

NOTE: The material contained in this book is set out in good
faith for general guidance and no liability can be accepted
for loss or expense incurred as a result of relying in particular
circumstances on statements made in the book. Laws and
regulations are complex and liable to change, and readers should
check the current position with the relevant authorities before
making personal arrangements.

Contents

8 Working as a Nurse

Preface

Until I started to do the research for this book, I had no idea how many options were open to nurses today. My co-writer, a practising nurse, and I have talked to a number of individuals who work in different fields. We have spoken to the matron of a hospice, an occupational therapist, a midwife, a social worker and a nursery nurse among others.

While maintaining an easy-to-read style, we have tried to make the book as comprehensive as possible. There are sections on working in a hospital, in the community, setting up your own nursing business, working abroad and many more.

For anyone who is contemplating a career in nursing or considering returning to nursing, we hope this book will provide a valuable insight into the training required for the various options and the wide range of opportunities that exist for prospective nurses. We have also included a chapter on other careers which are closely related to nursing.

Each chapter concludes with a case study. This provides an interesting and useful example of the daily life of the nurse and those who work alongside. Where names of staff and patients are used and experiences described, they are purely fictitious.

Marion Field

Acknowledgements

The authors would like to thank the following for their help in the compiling of this book:

Judy Affleck	Matron at a boarding school
Nicola Ayers	RGN (Registered General Nurse)
	Staff nurse at a boarding school
Kate Barrington	RGN (Registered General Nurse)
	DN (District Nurse)
Kate Downer	BSc (Hons) OT (Occupational Therapist)
	Occupational Therapist
Colin Edward	The Nursing Adviser to the Prison Service
Margaret Etheridge	SRN (State Registered Nurse)
	NNEB (National Nursery Exam. Board)
Simon Etheridge	Qualified Ambulance Technician
Bridget Forshaw	NNEB (National Nursery Exam. Board)
Linda Hicken	RGN (Registered General Nurse)
	RM (Registered Midwife)
Fran Law	RGN (Registered General Nurse)
	Diploma in Research Methodology
	Diploma in Nursing
	Diploma in Using Information
Liz Salter	RGN (Registered General Nurse)
	RMN (Registered Mental Nurse)
	BA (Hons)
	Counselling Diploma
Margaret Staunton-Lambert	SRN (State Registered Nurse)
	RCNT (Registered Clinical Nurse Tutor)
Stella Tassell	RGN (Registered General Nurse)
	RM (Registered Midwife)
	RMN (Registered Mental Nurse)
	RHV (Registered Health Visitor)
Liz Watkins	Diploma in Social Work
Marguerite Watts	RGN (Registered General Nurse)
	DN (District Nurse)
	Diploma in Palliative Care
	Matron at a hospice

The Woking Careers Office
The Woking Jobcentre

1

Finding Out About Nursing

Nursing is one of the most worthwhile jobs you can do. What could be more rewarding than easing the pain of a seriously ill patient, helping a child to walk again after an accident or teaching someone with a learning disability a new skill? These are only some of the useful tasks you might perform as a trained nurse.

MAKING THE RIGHT DECISION

How will you know if nursing is right for you? If you want to help people and are prepared to work hard, there is a wide variety of work you could do. If you are a school leaver, you may have done some work experience in a hospital or in some field related to nursing. That would be valuable experience.

Perhaps you wish to start a second career or you may want to enter nursing after having brought up your family. You could contribute a great deal to the profession by bringing to it your experience of either another career or bringing up a family.

Here are some of the **skills** you may need as a nurse:

- tact and sympathy

- organising skills

- the ability to work with and communicate well with other people

- calmness under pressure

- the ability to think clearly and solve problems.

Don't worry if you don't possess all of these at the moment; your training will help you to develop them.

Talking to people

Talk to any nurses you know and find out as much as you can about the work they do. If you don't know any, contact your local hospital and ask if you can visit and talk to some of the nurses. Have you ever had to visit the nurse who works with your local GP? She may be willing to give you some information and suggest some helpful journals you might read.

Ask your family and your teachers for their opinions. Do they feel nursing is the right career for you?

Going to the careers office
If you are still at school, you will probably have a careers teacher who may be able to give you appropriate information and will be able to discuss your future career and guide you in the right direction.

Your local careers office will also be helpful. Everything that is issued by the Department of Health is stored on file or on computer. A friendly assistant will help you find what you require. Ask if you could have a photocopy or print out of the particular documents that interest you.

Working as a volunteer
It is always useful to obtain 'hands on' experience before embarking on your training. If you are still at school, you would be very welcome as a volunteer in a hospital or nursing home. The hospital library often uses volunteers to distribute books and volunteers often visit the wards trundling the 'shop trolley'. You might be able to work at the weekends or during school holidays. It would also be useful to do some voluntary work after you have left school and before you start your training. The more experience you get, the more valuable it will be.

Writing to the colleges
If you are serious about taking up nursing as a career, you must decide on the type of training you require. Find out the addresses of those universities that have colleges of nursing attached to them. Your careers teacher, the careers office or your local library will be able to give you these.

Write to all those that are in a suitable area for you. Ask them to send you details of the nursing training they offer. There will be two main types – a diploma course known as Project 2000 and a degree course. These will be explained in more detail in Chapter 2.

LOOKING AT THE OPTIONS

Project 2000 consists of two parts. The first is called the Common Foundation and the second, the Branch Programme. You will have to choose your nursing speciality for the latter. There are four options, which are detailed below.

Choosing adult nursing

If you choose to train for adult nursing, you will have plenty of variety. Your patients will be suffering from a wide range of physical illnesses. You will work on a hospital ward, in an outpatient department, and an intensive care unit. You will care for elderly patients as well as young ones.

Nursing today is highly technical as the profession makes use of new technology. Once you are trained you will find you are given more responsibility for your patients. You no longer have to work directly under the direction of doctors and ward sisters. You will be able to plan the care your patient needs. In doing so, you must take account not only of their physical condition; it is important that you are familiar also with the patient's emotional, social and domestic situation as well.

Communication skills are very important as you will have to work in a team and give explanations and reassurance to your patients. You will have to assess your patients' needs and monitor their progress. Having done so, you should then know which other health care professionals you may need to call upon. You will experience nursing in the community and spend time with a district nurse, a health visitor or a specialist nurse.

Working with children

If you choose to be a children's nurse, you will be trained to work with boys and girls from birth to adolescence. You will learn about the physical and emotional development of children. Because your patients will not always be able to explain their symptoms, you will be trained to observe closely their behaviour as well as their medical condition. You will learn about community care, medical and surgical nursing and you will also deal with children with physical and learning disabilities, although specialist nurses will usually care for the latter.

You will work both in a hospital and in the community. Within the community you will work with a team of health care professionals. When dealing with children in hospital, you will require a high degree of **patience** and great **sympathy** as they are likely to be frightened by their environment. Your job will be to make it 'safe' for them.

As children now stay in hospital for shorter periods, you are likely to spend some of your training in the community. As well as caring for the child, you will also be involved with the parents, who are encouraged to play an active role in their children's care. You should gain their confidence and provide comfort and reassurance.

Working with children can be a rewarding experience particularly as you watch them recover their natural exuberance.

Helping those with learning disabilities

Learning disability nursing involves both care and practical skills. If you choose this branch of nursing, your role will be to help your patients achieve as much as possible.

You may have to teach very basic skills like washing and dressing. You will find that your patient can only absorb a little at a time and you will need a great deal of patience; you must give encouragement at every stage. If your patient is physically handicapped, you are likely to work with occupational therapists and physiotherapists.

You will work in a variety of different settings. The patient may live at home, be hospitalised, live in a hostel or even in a special community. Most of your work is likely to be in the community rather than in a hospital setting.

Opting for mental health nursing

There are many types of mental health problems and in your training you will deal with people of all ages who have different problems. Some will have serious mental problems which are enduring while others may suffer for only a short time – perhaps as a result of some trauma in their lives. Some patients will be cared for in rehabilitation centres while others will be in their home setting. Some will need to be in hospital for varying periods of time.

You will be trained in all aspects of mental health and will learn about the latest treatments. However, much of your work will consist of talking to and listening to your patients. It is important to build a relationship of trust with both them and their families.

SELECTING YOUR TRAINING

Now you have to decide what type of training you wish to do. Will you opt for a degree or for the diploma Project 2000? Both of these will be discussed in depth in the next chapter.

Applying for a course

For a place on the diploma course, you should write to: Nursing and Midwifery Admissions Service (NMAS), Fulton House, Jessop Avenue, Cheltenham GL50 3SH. You will be sent an application package including a handbook which gives details of courses. Applications should be in by December.

For a degree course you would apply through UCAS as for any other degree. The address is the same as the one above.

If you are interested in becoming a midwife, your training will be different from that of a nurse. Training to be a midwife will be dealt with in Chapter 8.

CHECKLIST

- Talk to people about your future.

- Use the careers office.

- Work as a volunteer.

- Find out about the courses.

CASE STUDY

Lucy makes her decision

Lucy is in her final school year. She is taking Biology and Chemistry at A level. She had always wanted to nurse and during the summer holidays she sent for the comprehensive application package from NMAS. She went to the library to obtain the addresses of appropriate universities which had a college of nursing attached to them. Her local careers office has been very helpful. She has filed for future reference the details about the variety of nursing she could do.

As she is taking A levels, her careers teacher at school feels she should apply to take a degree. But Lucy feels that the Project 2000 course might suit her better.

During the summer holidays she worked as a volunteer at a residential home for elderly people. The manager told her that she has a definite rapport with the clients.

'She told me I'll make a good nurse,' Lucy told her parents.

She knows she has to make a decision and during the autumn term she decides to apply for the Project 2000 course through NMAS. She is relieved she has made the decision and can now concentrate on her A levels.

2

Training to Be a Nurse

CHOOSING YOUR COURSE

There are two ways you can qualify as a **registered nurse.** You may choose to study for the diploma through the course known as Project 2000 or you may prefer to take a degree. Whichever you choose you will study at a college of nursing affiliated to a university.

INTRODUCING PROJECT 2000

Project 2000 is an exciting scheme. Before it was introduced, trainee nurses were expected to take on full nursing duties while on practical placements in hospital and the community. While there, they were expected to pass practical assessments as well as study for their exams. Project 2000 students continue to experience practical placements but their supernumerary status as students is more recognised. Now they are students just as in any other type of college or university. This means fairly long holidays and all the usual perks of student life.

The grant isn't brilliant, but it's adequate at about £4,572 per annum in 1999. Table 1 contains the pay scales for nurses and midwives.

Table 1: Whitley Pay Scales for Nurses and Midwives (April 1999) All scales have yearly increments.		
Grade D	Newly qualified nurse	£14,400 – £15,905
Grade E	Experienced nurse	£15,905 – £17,830
Grade F	Senior nurse	£17,830 – £20,925
Grade G	Sister/charge nurse	£20,925 – £23,300
Grade H	Senior sister/charge nurse	£23,300 – £25,735
Grade I	Clinical Nurse Manager	£25,735 – £28,240

Getting the right qualifications

To get into the Diploma course, Project 2000, you will need a minimum of five GCSEs at grade C or above or the equivalent. Some colleges of nursing have additional requirements so you will need to check this when you apply.

Taking the DC Test

If you don't have the appropriate qualifications required, don't despair. Some colleges of nursing offer an alternative. This is specially useful for older applicants who may not have had the opportunity to obtain GCSEs. Sometimes evidence of recent studying is required. You might have taken a BTEC course or studied at evening class.

This alternative is called the DC test. It is a timed test of one and a quarter hours consisting of English, verbal reasoning and maths. The minimum pass mark is 51 per cent but some nursing colleges require a higher one.

You are allowed three attempts at this test. The paper on each occasion will, of course, be different.

Working with the Common Foundation

The three year diploma course (Project 2000) is composed of two equal components – the Common Foundation and the Branch Programme.

The first 18 months are devoted to the Common Foundation which all Project 2000 students have to complete. This will equip you with the skills you will require for working with people both in hospital and in the community.

Every nursing college organises the course in a different way but there will probably be an introductory week followed by four terms of ten weeks each. A generous amount of time is allocated for study and holidays.

The introductory week

This is an exciting time; you will meet new colleagues, many of whom will become real friends as you go through your training. You will share many happy experiences. But you will also share some of the deep and painful experiences you are bound to meet – death, chronic illness, accidents. You will need each other, so take time to get to know your colleagues well. To help this, at the start of this week there are often 'ice breaking exercises' which encourage you to become better acquainted with those in your group and your tutors.

During this introductory week you will be given details about the whole course. You will be shown what is expected of you and given guidelines for assignments and projects and an outline of your practical placements.You will also hear talks from a variety of people who have important roles to play in the efficient working of the hospital and community services.

A fire officer is often the highlight of the week as you are introduced to the horrors of fire in a hospital setting. This talk often includes a practical element. For example, you may be ushered into a smoke-filled room and then expected to find your way out. The smoke is very disorientating and this sounds much easier than it is. Alternatively, you may just practise using the different types of fire extinguishers. Other speakers may include a union representative, a hospital chaplain and a hospital manager.

At the end of the week, you will have a much better understanding of the other professions you will be working with.

The first term
The pattern of work may vary but you will spend some time during the first term in the lecture hall concentrating on the theory of nursing practice and you will also go out on community visits. These visits are usually fun and may include time at a drop-in centre, a swimming pool, an ambulance station, a charity shop and Mcdonalds!

The following three terms
In the following terms you will spend three days each week studying nursing related subjects like anatomy, physiology, psychology, health promotion, causes of disease and its treatment and communication skills. The other two days – each of which is an eight hour shift – are spent getting 'hands on' experience out in the community and in a variety of hospital wards and departments.

Deciding on the Branch Programme
The second part of Project 2000 is the Branch Programme. Remember you can choose from adult nursing, children's nursing, learning disability nursing and mental health nursing. Training, of course, varies according to the speciality chosen. Details of these can be found in Chapter 1.

Gaining experience
You will be amazed at how quickly you become part of the hospital team. The wonderful thing about nursing is the variety of work opportunities offered and the different people you meet. As you gain experience, you will discover where you are most at home and can use your particular talents. Having gained sufficient experience, you may wish to undertake more specialist training to enable you to take on extra responsibility and to equip you for a higher grade. If you are a person who likes change, nursing means the world really is your oyster!

WORKING FOR YOUR DEGREE

If you wish to achieve a higher level of academic qualifications while studying to be a nurse, then the three or four year degree course might suit you. During this time you will engage in seminars, undertake small group tasks, produce project work and give presentations. You will also have the opportunity to gain practical experience. Theory will always be consolidated by practice.

Obtaining the prerequisite qualifications

For most courses you should have obtained a minimum of five GCSE passes at Grade C or above. It is hoped you will have received good grades in Maths, English and Science. (If you are a mature student, the equivalent of O levels will usually be accepted, but you should check with the appropriate university.) You should also possess one of the following:

● Two A level passes at Grade C or above. One of these should be a biological science.

● A two year full time or part time equivalent BTEC.

● Advanced GNVQ (General National Vocational Qualification).

If you have attended courses which are accredited to a university, you can acquire a number of points at various levels. These may count as credits towards your degree and, if so, will exempt you from taking certain modules.

If you already have a degree in a health-related subject, it may be possible for you to apply for an accelerated programme. It would normally take you two years to complete the course.

Your application could also be helped if you have learnt from a relevant practical experience in your own life. You might have cared for a dying parent, experienced a difficult birth or worked overseas. This is known as Accreditation for Prior Experiential Learning (APEL) and you may have the chance to demonstrate your knowledge either in an essay or at an interview. Obtain advice from the university about this.

Studying the modules

During your course you will cover a wide range of subjects. These may include subjects such as the history of nursing, research methods, sociology and psychology. Each block of work is called a module. A module consists of an approximate number of hours spent on a particular number of subjects. The modules are divided into various academic levels. To obtain your degree you have to complete a certain number of modules at each level. If you are unable to complete all of them, you may still have done enough to obtain your diploma.

Each module will be continuously assessed. The assessment may take a variety of forms. You will probably find coursework is an important element but you may also be expected to produce essays, projects, dissertations and also to sit examinations.

As you progress through your course, your pass marks will accumulate credits which will contribute to the classification of your degree.

Writing your essay

Make sure your essay is the best you can make it. Don't be satisfied with a first draft; do research and plan it thoroughly. Keep to the set number of words. You don't have to be exact but if you are asked for an essay of 3000 words, don't write 6000. You won't achieve a higher grade and will only annoy your tutor. You may be asked to rewrite it. One thousand words instead of 3000 is equally unacceptable but a variation of a hundred either way would be accepted. You will be provided with a brief outline plan of what is required and the marks that will be awarded.

Researching your work

Your research is very important. Make sure your facts are accurate and up-to-date. Become familiar with the libraries at the university and don't be afraid to ask the librarian for help if you require it. Make sure you keep a list of all the books you have used and include this bibliography at the end. It is also useful to make a separate list of specific references you have made. If you quote, you must acknowledge your source.

Planning your work

Having researched thoroughly, plan your work carefully deciding where each section best fits. It is often helpful to use subtitles. Do make sure you keep to the title and don't wander off the point or include a lot of irrelevant padding.

Producing the drafts

The way you write your essay is important. You are working for a degree so make sure your English is accurate and you haven't sprinkled your work with commas instead of full stops!

After completing your first draft, go through it *very* carefully, correcting and adjusting it. Does it make sense? Does it contain what you want to say? Is it the right length? It is often helpful to ask a friend to read your work before submitting it.

Revising the points

● Research thoroughly.

● Plan your essay carefully.

● Check it.

● Keep to the required length.

Preparing your dissertation

You will usually have to prepare and present a final dissertation. This can be a subject of your own choice and is often a topic about which little has been written. However, you will be expected to make reference to supporting published research so avoid a subject which doesn't have any. Your choice of subject may be related to a particular aspect of nursing care in which you have an interest. This could be the care of leg ulcers in the elderly, or the communication needs of children in hospital.

Perhaps something more managerial may interest you. For example you may wish to question the relevance of a policy or procedure: should families be asked to leave the bedside of their loved one at a cardiac arrest emergency? Detailed discussion with your tutor should take place before you start on your work.

Use your practical work to support your views and be ready to justify from practical experience the points you have made. If you find you disagree with something you have read or been told, support your views by examples. If you can't do so, you are probably wrong!

Sitting your exam

If you have to sit an exam, don't panic! Here are some guidelines:

● Plan your revision over several weeks.

● Don't leave all your revising until the night before!

● Get enough sleep so you are not too tired.

● Plan your time before you start writing the paper and try not to overrun on the first question.

Choosing your option

The four main branches of nursing have been detailed in Chapter 1. They are: adult nursing, children's nursing, learning disability nursing and mental health nursing. For your degree you can specialise in one of them although you will obviously also study related subjects.

FOCUSING ON NVQ

The National Vocational Qualification would be ideal for you if you want to nurse but don't want the commitment of studying as intensively as in the above trainings.

The NVQ certificate can be studied at your own pace. There are no minimal entry requirements. You will have an assessor who will help you to gather all the evidence you need to prove your understanding and efficiency in each unit. This is a fairly new training in nursing and is still being changed to improve its effectiveness. It is work-based but you will also be expected to produce a high standard of written work. There are no examinations and the pace is as fast or as slow as you wish to make it. At various intervals you are expected to undertake short training sessions in the classroom to give you the necessary knowledge. This usually happens in the training department in your place of work. If you want to work as a care assistant, levels two and three are most appropriate but there are higher levels for those with management responsibilities. A word of warning – some employers may ask for a contribution towards the cost of an NVQ award, especially if you have not been working with them for long.

Working as a care assistant

It is still possible to work as a care assistant without any formal training in hospital and the community but you will find that most good and caring establishments are encouraging their staff to take the NVQ course. Once you have completed the course, you will have a better understanding of why you nurse the way you do and you will have developed certain skills. This training will help you to experience rewarding and satisfying work.

LIVING AS A NURSE

You will find many changes in your life style as you start your nursing training; some are good and some not so good, but most of them will be interesting.

Enjoying the uniform

Nurses' uniform has changed radically over the years. For male nurses it has tended to become more comfortable and less starchy! For female nurses, the change is more noticeable. You may find yourself in a tunic top and trousers rather than the traditional dress and apron. Few hospitals still expect nurses to wear a cap except as a genuine head covering when, for example, working in the theatre.

Grades of seniority are usually denoted by the colour of your belt; this, too, varies in each hospital. Some nurses, particularly those who work in the mental heath sector and the community, usually only wear identity badges and not a uniform.

Long, loose hair is not acceptable for hygienic reasons. Changing dressings with hair hanging over the wound is obviously wrong.

Your feet will walk many miles on the wards and they will appreciate comfortable, 'sensible' shoes; you might not like the look of them but you will soon appreciate the comfort!

Finding accommodation

You will be glad to know that the days have gone when nurses were expected to live in nurses' homes and had to be in their rooms by ten o'clock most nights. Nowadays hospital accommodation is in short supply and you will probably have to find your own 'digs'. There are usually plenty of places suitable for students around the larger hospitals – houses divided into bed-sits or shared flats for those who like more company. Some colleges of nursing also offer accommodation.

You might be offered hospital accommodation and this is well worth considering. Although not cheap, it is usually of a high standard. Meals can be bought as you want them and are varied and interesting. If this is your first experience of living away from home, you may have a few problems coming to terms with being responsible for paying the bills, doing the cleaning and remembering to keep enough food in the fridge! But the pleasures far outweigh the problems.

Enduring or enjoying shifts

There are three main shifts, though of course this varies in different hospitals. Most shifts are eight hours long although some hospitals are now experimenting with a twelve hour shift rota. You will eventually be included in the duty rota and will be expected to rotate your shifts so that everyone has a fair share of days and nights. You may find shifts strange and difficult to cope with at first, but they will soon become just another part of your life.

The early shift usually starts at 7.30 and finishes at 15.30. Although not so good after a late night, this shift is popular because it leaves the afternoon and evening free to do your own thing. The late shift starts at 14.00 and ends at 22.00.

The night shift is not so socially acceptable as it starts at 21.15 and ends at 7.30. You may find you have extra difficulty in adjusting to it. Going to work when everyone else is going out for the evening can be very frustrating and having your breakfast when your friends are having their supper is a strange experience. You might find it difficult to sleep during the day, especially if you have noisy neighbours.

However, there are lots of advantages. You can do your shopping peacefully in crowd-free stores, sleep in the garden when others are working in a stuffy office and because you work longer hours on consecutive nights, your off-duty mounts up and can seem like a mini-holiday. Night duty has a very special feeling for many nurses and it is an experience you will probably enjoy. Nurses on night duty and those working after 20.00 hours usually earn more money.

BELONGING TO A TRADE UNION

During your training you will be encouraged to join a trade union. This provides you with indemnity and other services. Most nurses belong to one of the following:

● Royal College of Nursing (RCN)

● UNISON (an amalgamation of NUPE, COHSE and NALGO).

Finding opportunities with the RCN

The RCN is the union closest to the nursing profession. The officials are all nurses voted into their positions by the members who provide views on proposed policies and suggest new services the RCN can offer. As a member, you are entitled to give your views to your local steward or you might be interested in becoming the RCN steward for your region. You have, therefore, the opportunity to influence the RCN's policy on nursing matters. Through attending the annual RCN Congress, you will be able to:

● participate in study activities

● meet old and new acquaintances

● learn more about services offered

● listen to and question international nursing leaders

● visit the exhibition which features the latest nursing products, job opportunities and services.

Other services provided by the RCN

● legal and professional advice

● RCN Internet website (www.rcn.org.uk.)

- grants and bursaries
- research project opportunities
- forums for different nursing fields
- national and local conferences and study days
- nursing journals, books, leaflets and circulars
- information and support on new nursing issues
- negotiation with the government on matters relating to nursing
- workshops on implementation of new government legislation
- campaigning for better working conditions
- guidelines on clinical practice.

In addition the RCN has links with many organisations which can provide RCN members with discount rates for various services:

- car sales
- RAC membership
- holidays
- insurance
- endowment policies
- clothes discounts
- RCN Visa card.

KEEPING UP TO DATE

Every practising nurse, midwife and health visitor has to be registered with the governing body, the **United Kingdom Central Council (UKCC)**. To maintain this registration you must fulfil the requirements of Post Registration Education and Practice (PREP) as laid down by the UKCC.

Finding out about PREP

PREP aims to increase your knowledge and to develop the skills you will need in order to practise competently. By encouraging you to keep up to date with changes in your area of nursing, PREP ensures that high standards of nursing care for your patients are maintained. To demonstrate this you must keep a **Personal Professional Profile** (PPP).

The PREP requirements
To keep up your PREP requirements you must:

- re-register by completing a **notification of practice form** every three years

- do the equivalent of five days of study every three years

- keep a Personal Professional Profile (PPP) which illustrates your professional development

- complete a **Return to Practice** course if you have worked less than 750 hours or 100 days in the five years preceding re-registration.

Notification of practice
The UKCC will notify you 45 days before your registration is due to expire. You will be sent a notification of practice form which will list all your qualifications and ask you which you are using in your current practice. You will have to specify your current work area.

Study days
The health care environment is constantly changing. In order to keep up to date with the changes, you must develop your knowledge and skills so that a high standard is maintained. PREP requires you to do the equivalent of five days of study every three years. You can fulfil this requirement in a variety of ways:

- attend a conference or seminar

- take a course

- visit other departments

- undertake individual study

- take a correspondence course

- attempt project work with your colleagues.

Before deciding on your area of study and the way you will do it, the UKCC PREP document (*PREP and you*, published by UKCC) recommends you ask yourself some relevant questions to help your decision making. Your study, of course, must be related to your current area of practice.

Here are some questions:

- What are your strong and weak points?

● In which areas do you need to develop your skills?

● What do you aim to achieve?

● Do you need to ask for study time? Discuss it with your manager before you confirm your study activities.

When you have completed your study requirements, ask yourself some more questions:

● What did you learn?

● Did you achieve your goals?

● Did your study help you to meet your patients' needs?

● How can you share what you have learnt with your colleagues?

● How can you incorporate what you have learnt into your personal professional profile?

Keeping a Personal Professional Profile (PPP)

The UKCC has not stipulated the pattern the PPP should take but the content should reflect your personal professional development. Through reflecting on your study activities and writing about its application to your work you can demonstrate how you have met the PREP requirements for study. A PPP is not a CV or a diary but a flexible catalogue of your career and learning achievements. It serves to:

● remind you of what you have learnt and accomplished

● remind you of dates, jobs and courses you have taken

● enable you to reflect on past learning experiences that will help you plan for the future.

Writing your profile

To help you organise your Personal Professional Profile (PPP) the UKCC and the Royal College of Nursing (RCN) regularly provide study days on the topic. You will find advertisements for these in the nursing press, on hospital notice boards and in inservice training departments. The following information should be included in your PPP:

● biographical details

● professional and academic qualifications

● details of employment

- areas of professional practice you would like to develop
- a record of your learning objectives and how you have achieved them
- certificates of attendance at study sessions
- a record of your recent employment.

Always apply what you have learnt to your work. By doing this and by documenting it in your PPP you have fulfilled the requirements of PREP and ensured that your nursing care is up to date. You can keep up to date in a variety of ways:

- reading nursing and medical journals
- surfing the Internet
- project work by yourself or with colleagues
- attending nursing study days or conferences
- attending courses run by the hospital training department
- attending seminars
- attending regional nurses' meetings
- correspondence courses
- visiting other departments and hospitals
- discussing a case study with your colleagues.

Applying for a course

With your application form for a course, you may have to submit an essay on a given title. Look back in this chapter for some information on writing essays.

Preparing for the interview

Because so many nurses apply to attend courses, you may have to attend an interview before being accepted on to some. At the interview be confident about your abilities and convince the interviewing panel that you would benefit from the course and use what you will learn in your daily practice. You may be in competition with many other candidates so the interviewers will have a difficult task ahead of them. Why should they choose you instead of another good candidate?

Presenting your experience
Don't be shy to speak about yourself. Talk about areas in which you have an interest, courses you have already taken and relevant experience you have had. Read through your Personal Professional Profile to remind yourself of how much you have achieved. Refresh your memory about the PREP requirements. Tell the panel what journals you regularly read and what you are currently studying. Convince the interviewers that you are committed to improving patient care and are interested in increasing your management skills. Don't be afraid to indicate your future career hopes. Make sure you are up to date with current Health Service issues.

Questions you may be asked

- Why have you chosen this course?

- Will you be able to cope with its demands?

- How will you benefit from it?

- Have you already had experience in this area?

- Will you be able to use what you learn in your daily practice?

- What are your future plans?

Returning to Practice

If you have worked for less than 750 hours or 100 days during a five year period, this constitutes a break in practice. To re-register you would have to complete successfully a Return to Practice programme. This would be at least five days long and would include a period of supervised practice. You will learn more about this in Chapter 10.

CHECKLIST

- Details of Project 2000 and degree.

- Prerequisite requirements.

- Information about NVQ.

- Life as a nurse.

- Keeping up to date.

- Checking PREP and PPP.

CASE STUDY

A night in the life of Anne, a student nurse

Anne is coming to the end of her training as a Registered General Nurse on the Project 2000 course. Currently she is doing night duty in a female surgical ward. It is Saturday evening.

Anne's diary

Why did I have to be on night duty tonight of all nights? It was Kate's wedding today and I'd been looking forward to it for ages but I kept looking at my watch wondering how much longer I dare stay. I left it as late as I could and then took a taxi to the hospital sucking mints all the way to cover up the smell of drink – not that I'd drunk very much but I didn't want to smell of alcohol while on duty!

Of course, by the time I'd changed I was late on the ward and Sue and Pat were already taking the report from the day staff. Pat, the health care assistant, started on the drinks while I started to do the 'obs' (observations), (temperature, pulse and blood pressure). Then I checked the drips. Most of the patients had some kind of drip, infusion pump, drain or catheter as it was a surgical ward. Thankfully, tonight was a Saturday so no new routine operations had been admitted.

I hadn't got very far when Mrs West started calling out for a bed pan. Of course that set all the patients off. Pat and I were rushing round trying to be in five places at once as we distributed bed pans and commodes.

As soon as 'bed pan alley' had subsided, I went back to checking the 'obs' and 'drips'. Mrs Brown's drip of normal saline had gone through too slowly. It was supposed to go in over eight hours and at least a third was still left after that time. I checked her blood pressure and then speeded up the drip. I planned to tell Sue, the senior nurse, when I saw her.

Just as I thought I could sit down to a cup of coffee, Sue called me to help with the medicines. They took ages because they have to be checked so carefully. I remembered to tell Sue about Mrs Brown's drip.

We'd just managed to take a few sips of coffee when there was a bump and a loud moan. Mrs White had fallen out of bed. She said she'd been trying to rearrange the bed clothes. Pat and I made her comfortable on the floor while Sue went to bleep Dr Gibbs. He came quickly and examined her and said we could put her back to bed. I went to get the hoist and sling equipment we'd just acquired. As I wheeled it down from the bathroom, the squeaky wheels woke up all the other patients. Consequently, we had another 'bed pan alley' run and then at last we sat down at the nurses' station for that much needed cup of coffee and Sue filled out an accident form for Mrs White.

I was relieved when it was one o'clock and I could go to the dining room for a meal. I wasn't very hungry but it was pleasant to sit down for a while. I don't usually like walking down the long corridors at night but Jane, another student, was also on nights so we walked over together.

The rest of the night was fairly quiet although poor Mrs White kept ringing her bell. I sat with her for a while and this seemed to help her to get to sleep. By the time the day staff came on duty at half past seven I was shattered. Much as I love 'nights', I couldn't wait to collapse into bed to dream of my nights off!

3

Working in a Hospital

When you are a trained nurse, you might choose to work in a hospital. As you are newly qualified, you will find it useful to work on the wards initially to get some basic nursing experience. After this, you may want to stay where you are, specialise or branch into other areas within the hospital. You might be interested in management, teaching or research.

COMBINING THEORY WITH PRACTICE

The theory you have learnt needs to be put into practice. Much of what you do as a nurse is based on feelings of sympathy, empathy, compassion and your want to care. However, in addition to this your work is based on theories and research. As you apply the theories you have learnt and continue to be aware of the research in your field, your nursing will remain up to date and your care the best for your patient.

Many hospitals help their nurses to apply theory and research to their practice by providing **manuals of care**, often in the form of written standards or procedures. You will find them in each ward or department. A practice development nurse based in the hospital will help you to keep them up to date.

WORKING ON THE WARDS

As a ward based nurse, you will experience both enjoyable and stressful times which will be shared with a team of nurses. The other nurses will become friends who will help if you experience difficulties. Stress may come if you are short staffed or if there is an emergency to test your skills and knowledge. All your experiences will help you to develop your skills and face future challenges with confidence.

Becoming a staff nurse

You will never forget the day you walk on to the ward wearing your staff nurse's uniform for the first time. You will feel jubilation mixed with fear because, as a qualified nurse, you are now accountable for your actions. Don't worry! You will not be expected to work without support. For the first four months you will be helped to achieve certain objectives by an experienced colleague. This 'preceptorship' period is demanded by the nursing governing body which has laid down this requirement in the Post Registration Education Practice document (PREP).

Working in a surgical unit

If you work on a surgical unit you may either stay on one ward or rotate around the unit. By rotating you will have plenty of variety. Smaller hospitals may have one surgical ward doing varied operations. Larger hospitals tend to have more surgical wards with each one specialising in treating patients who have a problem with a specific area of their bodies.

Specialist surgical wards

- Gynaecology ward – female patients needing operations on the urinary and genital tract.

- Urology ward – patients needing operations on the urinary system.

- Gastroenterology ward – patients needing stomach or bowel operations.

- Orthopaedic ward – patients needing bone or joint operations.

- ENT ward – patients needing operations on ears, nose or throat.

Whether you work on a general or specialist ward much of your work will be the same. You will have to prepare patients for their operations and care for them when they return to the ward.

Preparing your patient for the operation

The physical care of your patients before the operation will include the following:

- bathing them

- storing their belongings safely

- administering pre-medication

- taking a heart reading (ECG)

- helping them with an X-ray

- taking blood samples.

The emotional care of your patients before they go to the theatre may include the following:

- explaining the operation and its after effects
- listening to their anxieties and answering their questions
- talking to their families
- arranging visits from social workers
- addressing their spiritual needs.

Caring for the patients after the operation
After the operation, the emotional care continues and the physical care becomes more intense. It is likely there will be some intravenous infusions (drips). You must make sure that these are given as prescribed by the doctor. You will also have to assess how effective they are. Is the medication helping to relieve the pain? Ask the patient to grade the pain on a scale of one to ten so that you can judge whether the pain relief should be increased or decreased.

You will find the work challenging but rewarding as you watch your patients' health improve because of the care you have given them.

Experiencing a medical ward

Working on a medical ward is very different from working on a surgical ward. Medical patients are often in hospital for a long time so you will get to know them and their visitors very well. They will often require much more basic nursing care and will need help to wash, dress, eat and exercise. Many will have problems which will take a long time to overcome. As well as your basic nursing skills you will also need skills to educate, rehabilitate and empathise; you may be required to help them re-learn simple tasks they have been doing all their lives. They may have diabetes or have had a bad fall. They may also be suffering from any of the following:

- pneumonia
- asthma
- a stroke
- heart failure
- eating disorders
- uncontrolled skin condition (*eg* leg ulcer or psoriasis).

Using other professionals
There are other professionals who will help you in the care of your patients. They include:

- physiotherapist

- occupational therapist

- speech therapist

- hospital chaplain

- diabetic specialist nurse

- social worker

- dietician.

Caring for your patients
Many of your patients will have come straight from home and some are likely to be elderly and in poor health. They may have been trying to cope alone for a long time. As well as treating their medical problems, you will have to help them to build up their strength, confidence and their will to live.

Preparing for death
Sadly some of your patients will not live to see their homes again. Preparing your patients, their families and friends for death is a difficult part of your role. Nevertheless, you will find it rewarding when you can help your patient to experience a peaceful and dignified death. If you have not encountered death before, you may find it disturbing. The more experienced nurses on the ward and the hospital chaplain will help you to manage your feelings so that the next time it is less disturbing.

Your experience on a medical ward will be a fulfilling one and the skills you learn and develop will provide a solid foundation for the work you do during your nursing career.

Practising primary nursing

To comply with the Patients' Charter introduced by the Department of Health in 1991, **primary nursing** has been introduced. This ensures that a named qualified nurse, midwife or health visitor is responsible for each patient's care for the duration of his or her stay on the ward. The senior and junior nurses work in teams and a qualified nurse from each team acts as the primary nurse to an allocated group of patients.

Advantages of primary nursing

- The patient knows their named nurse.

- Patient and nurse communication can be improved.

- The patient's visitors can talk to a particular nurse.

- The patient's needs are better understood.

- The doctor can identify the primary nurse.

Disadvantages

- Caring for a very sick or difficult patient for a long period can be stressful so the standard of nursing care could be compromised.

- The opportunity to learn about other patients' conditions is limited.

- The continuity of care may be disturbed by the primary nurse's unavoidable absence.

Becoming a ward manager

After experience and progression within the field of your choice you may wish to become a ward manager (sister/charge nurse). In this position you will be the most senior nurse on the ward and therefore responsible for its management. The skills you have developed through experience and the courses you have completed will help you to fulfil the role.

Your responsibilities may also include the following:

- taking charge of the ward when on duty

- dealing with the budget for the ward

- attending managers' meetings

- planning the duty rota and ensuring there are enough nurses and the right grades on each shift

- reporting and dealing with problems – patient bed crisis, staff or patient accident, a violent or missing patient

- acting as adviser, teacher and role model for the rest of your staff

- appraising your staff and making sure they achieve learning objectives

- counselling individuals.

Managing your own ward can be a rewarding experience. It provides you with the opportunity to be innovative. Perhaps you may wish to introduce a new shift pattern – or primary nursing.

PROGRESSING IN YOUR FIELD

If you wish to progress but stay in the same field of nursing, you can apply for a higher grade post. Usually the minimum requirement for this is experience in that particular area. However, sometimes you are required to take a specialist course to update your knowledge. Your responsibilities will increase as you become more senior. They will include teaching students and junior staff and managing the ward in the absence of the sister or charge nurse. If you wish to continue on the promotion ladder, you may have to take courses that cover teaching and management skills.

If you have found your niche and do not want the increased responsibility that comes with promotion, progression for you may be reflecting on your experiences and keeping up to date with any changes in nursing. You will continue to improve your nursing care and self development.

CHOOSING TO BRANCH OUT

There may come a time when you wish to leave the ward but still work in the hospital. By keeping an eye on the job vacancies you will discover many new and exciting positions. It is a big step to leave the ward but you can always return. Experience in other nursing positions, even for a short time, will enhance your skills. Many hospitals offer seconded positions. These allow you to work in a new job for a specific length of time and then return to your previous post. Working for a short time in another post can help you decide if a change of scene is really what you need. Here are some of the possibilities:

- specialist nurse

- nurse practitioner

- nurse teacher

- patient representative

- nursing manager

- research nurse

- hospital occupational health nurse

- audit nurse.

Further training may be required for some of these. However, you may be offered the opportunity to train while in the post.

Working as a specialist nurse

A specialist nurse is an experienced nurse who has undertaken further training and developed additional skills in order to look after patients with specialised needs. If you choose this, your workplace will not be confined to one ward but you will be available to help patients and nurses in any department. This may include working in the community. Your role will include the physical and emotional care of the patient and a large proportion of teaching. Teaching skills are essential because it may be necessary to teach the patient how to manage a problem. You will also have to teach other staff how to help the patient and teach on training days. Here are some of the specialist nurse posts:

- infection control

- breast care

- respiratory care

- stoma care (caring for patients who have had abdominal surgery, often resulting from cancer)

- palliative care (alleviating some of the symptoms of the disease)

- incontinence.

Becoming a nurse practitioner

This is a new position for senior nurses who wish to develop the service they can offer their patients. At the time of writing in 1999 there are no agreed standards of training or practice. Instead, individual hospitals and nurses working in these posts decide on their own standards and guidelines of practice.

As a nurse practitioner, you could be employed in an accident and emergency department. Here you will assess the injury, decide what is wrong and treat and discharge patients with minor injuries. In this situation the patient does not see the doctor. Nurse practitioners are also working in the field of urology where they run clinics; they assess men with prostate problems, take and report on bladder tests and provide follow-up care including injections and counselling for patients who have prostate or bladder cancer.

This is an exciting post because, if its development remains focused on nursing care, the service you will offer your patients will be greatly enhanced.

Becoming a nurse teacher

As a staff nurse working in the hospital or in the community you will already be teaching other nurses but the opportunity exists for you to work as a nurse teacher. You should be an experienced nurse, preferably with a teaching qualification and degree. You could be based in an inservice training department of a hospital, a college of nursing or a clinical area in a hospital.

Teaching in an inservice training department

Many National Health Service Trusts have their own training departments. Within these are nurse teachers who teach a variety of courses for the nursing staff. You may also be required to teach at other venues including private nursing homes. Your role as a nurse teacher in a hospital would be to help other nurses develop their knowledge and improve their practice. You will work with a team of nurse teachers. You may be offered the post because of your experience but may be encouraged to undertake further training while in the post.

You will be teaching qualified nurses and those studying for National Vocational Qualifications (NVQ) throughout the hospital trust. You may also be required to teach in the community. Your teaching will be varied and at different levels. It will include simple anatomy and physiology, assertiveness, appraisal skills and management. Little time will be spent teaching on the wards as the nurses will visit your training department. However, if a specific problem should arise on the ward, then teaching on the ward may be necessary.

Working in a college

If you choose to work in a college, you will be teaching student nurses who are on the Project 2000 course or taking a degree; you may also be teaching qualified nurses undertaking post registration courses. You will have the challenge of teaching at many different educational levels. You may find the anatomy, physiology and history of nursing classes relatively simple, but the discussion following ethics seminars stimulating. Your role will be to provide information and guidance, facilitate self-directed learning and assess your students' progress. For most of the time you will be based in the college but at times you may be required to work with your students while they are on practical placements.

Teaching in a clinical area

If you are based in a clinical area, you will be referred to as a lecturer/ practitioner. For some of the time you will be performing nursing duties and the remaining time you will teach the nursing staff based in the area. You may also be required to teach outside the clinical area. These positions are very popular as they provide variety and stimulus.

Contact with the patients and the nursing team is maintained at the same time as your role of teacher and staff developer. An intensive care unit is likely to employ a lecturer/practitioner. New staff need comprehensive orientation and experienced staff need regular updating on new technology and new methods of working.

As a lecturer/practitioner, you will teach individuals as well as groups and organise group study days. As well as teaching about nursing issues, you will provide information, guidance and practice for job or course interviews. You may also be responsible for doing performance reviews for the nursing staff. To do a lecturer/practitioner's job satisfactorily you must be committed and prepared to work hard as the combined role is demanding and challenging. However, if you enjoy teaching and aiding the development of your colleagues as well as using your nursing skills, this job could be right for you.

Becoming a nursing manager

A nursing manager is an experienced nurse who has usually undertaken additional training including possibly a higher degree. The role varies between organisations and is constantly changing to meet the needs of the health service. Some managerial responsibilities have now been given to ward managers.

Taking responsibility

As a nursing manager, you will have overall responsibility for several departments. Your role will include:

● dealing with staff – shortlistings, interviews, suspensions and dismissals

● individual performance reviews

● budgeting

● management of changes

● negotiating between medical staff, nursing staff and administrative staff

● counselling individuals and supporting teams of nurses

- implementing local and government policy

- meeting long term goals

- crisis management – bed shortages, excessive staff sickness, patients' treatment.

You will usually work office hours and you may miss contact with patients. However, you can visit the wards regularly and introduce yourself to some of the patients. This will enable you to remain aware of how they feel and what improvements they would like to see.

Your role is primarily an administrative one. You will have to attend meetings and cope with a lot of paperwork. You must be competent at meeting deadlines. Although the pay is better than that of a ward nurse, the opportunity to earn more for weekends, nights or late duties is minimal. You may feel isolated as you are neither one of the 'workers' or one of the 'bosses', but you and your senior nurses can work towards pioneering nursing projects. You can expect to be paid either an H or an I grade.

Skills required by a nursing manager

- assertiveness

- ability to motivate others

- enthusiasm

- punctuality

- time management

- decision making

- negotiation skills

- good communication skills

- approachability

- ability to take responsibility

- presentation skills

- commitment.

Going into research

If you wish to undertake nursing research, you could be employed in an academic research environment but these opportunities are limited and remove you from the nursing field.

The position of research nurse in the hospital setting covers a multitude of different roles. You could be employed to undertake a research project connected with a specific area of nursing; you might be interested in the effectiveness of patient information supplied by nurses. This post would probably have conditions attached to it and be constrained by a budget. It is also likely to be for a set period of time. When completed, you may be required to present a strategy for change to practice if you found this to be necessary.

As a research nurse you could also take responsibility for the care of patients involved in clinical research trials. They may be taking new medication or trying out new devices. Your role would be to make sure the patient is well informed and well looked after during the trial. You will also have to ensure the trial runs smoothly and is in line with local, national and international standards. You may also have the opportunity to undertake your own nursing research in a subject of your choice.

Choosing research will offer you a challenge which is new, exciting and different. If this area of nursing interests you, find out if there are any research nurses employed at your hospital and have a chat with them.

UNDERTAKING FURTHER EDUCATION

If you complete the training necessary to achieve a senior nursing position but wish to continue with further education, you might consider taking a degree or studying for a teaching certificate. You might even choose to do a master's degree or a PhD. Higher education courses for nurses are becoming popular and are more accessible. However, you should consider doing the course on a part-time basis as the opportunity to study full time as a nurse is limited.

CHECKLIST

- Ask other nurses about their jobs.
- Don't be afraid to ask other members of staff for help.
- Talk with friends or relatives about their experiences as patients.
- Don't expect to know everything.
- Enjoy caring for your patients.
- Check the advertisements in the job bulletin.

CASE STUDY

A day in the life of a research nurse

Rachel enjoys her work as a research nurse; she works with a team of doctors, technicians, administrative staff and other nurses. Her work varies but on this particular morning she checks on her regular patients who are taking a new tablet for chest complaints. She chats with each of them, takes their blood pressure, a heart reading and a blood test. Dave, one of her patients, tells her about a rash he has noticed. She decides it could be a side effect of the tablets so she reports the details to the research doctor before allowing Dave to continue with the trial.

When she has completed her paperwork and informed Dave's GP about his problem, it is lunch time. She takes her sandwich to the lunchtime seminar on 'How to achieve the PREP requirements'.

After lunch she sees another patient, Sandra; Rachel and the research doctor explain about a new trial which may help her. Sandra and her husband discuss the new treatment but decide not to take part as regular visits to the department would be too inconvenient for them.

The second patient they see does agree to take part as they are very anxious to sort out their chest problem. Rachel and the doctor complete the tests which are required and arrange to see them again in one week's time.

Rachel has recently completed a course dealing with presentation and computer skills run by the training department of the hospital. She decides to put her presentation skills into practice. After checking that it is convenient, she visits the chest ward to brief the nurses about a new trial which would involve their patients. She is pleased with her presentation and delighted with the positive feedback she received about the handouts she provided.

She returns home to work on a poster she has been asked to prepare for a forthcoming national conference. She knows the skills she has recently acquired will be very useful.

4

Going into the Community

If you like plenty of variety and fewer restrictions on how you manage your working day, you might decide to follow a career outside the hospital. There are various options open to you.

WORKING AS A DISTRICT NURSE

District nursing started in 1859 when William Rathbone, a wealthy Liverpool shipowner, employed a nurse to look after his wife who was in the last stages of consumption (tuberculosis). So impressed was he with the care she provided that he asked her to set up a nursing organisation to look after the poor and the sick. He also contacted Florence Nightingale,who persuaded the Liverpool Infirmary to train its own nurses to send out into the community. District nursing was born and was considerably helped in 1887 when Queen Victoria donated some money to help with the training.

Training as a district nurse

To train as a district nurse, you must be a registered nurse and then work for the district nurse's degree which will take you one or two years. If you have already taken a four year degree course, you may receive some exemptions; however, if you did the Project 2000 diploma, you will be expected to do the whole course.

Liaising with other professionals

Once you are trained, you will usually work with a GP who will refer patients to you. However, you may also receive referrals from hospitals, the Social Services, a health visitor, a midwife, a school nurse or a specialist nurse working in the community. You will always work closely with other professionals to ensure the best care of your patients. You will usually work from 8.30 to 17.00 but will sometimes be expected to be on call to cover evenings and weekends with a nursing care service.

Working as a team

As a trained district nurse, you will lead a team which may include community staff nurses and community health care assistants. You will be responsible for planning and supervising the care the patients receive. To do this it will be necessary for you to visit and assess each patient to see what care is needed and which members of your team can best provide it. Perhaps after assessment, you may decide your patient needs a raised toilet seat or some other amenity.

Sometimes it will be necessary for you to enlist the help of other community workers. You may work with community specialist nurses like continence advisers or occupational therapists.

Treating the patients

Your patients will be anyone who needs nursing care in the home but they are likely to be mainly adult. You may have a number of frail, elderly people who need regular nursing care at home. Now that patients are discharged from hospital more quickly after an operation, they will need post operative care at home. It is your role to provide this. Patients who have had surgery will also require your help until they have fully recovered. Your aim will always be to provide care and support which will enable your patients to regain their independence.

Because you visit them in their homes, you are in a unique position to promote health through education in an informal way. This will be an important part of your work. As far back as 1883 Florence Nightingale remarked that nurses encouraged their patients to lead a healthy life style by their example. As well as providing nursing care and support for relatives, you may be able to alleviate any health hazards in the home and promote good health by your example and by discussing the problems. You can also encourage your patients to be aware of how to live a healthy life by bringing particular television documentaries and specific articles to their attention.

Some National Health Trusts now run care schemes called 'Hospital at Home'. This provides health care in the patient's home and offers more intensive care than can be offered by the usual community services. It is not relevant for patients who have long term health problems but is suitable for those who need short term care. Perhaps the patient has recently had a stroke or is recovering from a surgical operation.

Coping with a wide range of tasks

As a district nurse you may choose to specialise in a particular area but much of your work will be very varied. As well as needing care because of age or an operation, your patients may need care in the following areas:

● wound care

● pain control

● intravenous therapy (working with drips and blood transfusions)

● stoma care (caring for patients who have had abdominal surgery usually resulting from cancer)

● continence promotion (helping patients who are incontinent)

● phlebotomy (taking blood samples)

● HIV/AIDS

● drug and alcohol dependency

● physical disability

● severe learning disabilities

● dialysis (helping patients on kidney machines).

Skills required for district nursing

● assessment skills

● management skills

● communication skills

● awareness of up-to-date research

● the ability to teach by example

● a willingness to use the media to promote health education

● an awareness of the current social climate.

Assessing your pay

Rates of pay will vary depending on where you are working. As a qualified district nurse you can expect to be paid at least on an F grade but a G grade is more likely. As a community nurse new to the area, you would expect to start on a D grade and with district nursing experience you would progress to an E grade. You will earn more if you work unsocial hours – evening and weekends.

Revising the points

- You will work with a GP.

- You will visit patients in their own homes.

- You need management skills to run a team.

- You will promote a healthy life style.

WORKING AS AN OCCUPATIONAL HEALTH NURSE

If you choose to work as an occupational health nurse, you are advised to do some further training in this field. Courses are available at various colleges and universities and lists of the colleges offering the courses can be obtained from the Royal College of Nursing, 20 Cavendish Square, London W1M 0AB. When you are qualified, you will sometimes be invited to attend short courses, study days and conferences on specific topics.

Nursing in industry

If you work for a large industrial organisation, you may be involved in a variety of work.

Coping with health hazards

If there is a particular health hazard at the plant, you will be responsible for making sure employees are aware of it and are shown the best ways of avoiding infection or accidents. If workers have been exposed to constant dust, you will have to monitor them and carry out the necessary health screening. This may mean measuring their lung capacity on a regular basis. You may be asked to identify particular health hazards and find ways of reducing their danger. To encourage a 'safe' environment for the workers, you will probably have to work with safety officers.

Record keeping will be an important part of your job and you will be expected to keep a note of all accidents and illnesses which occur in case there is a recurring pattern. You will also have to record the results of any tests the employees have taken.

Dealing with employees

You may be one of the first people a prospective employee meets as a fitness test may be appropriate. If he or she is appointed, it is your role to make sure that safety regulations are known and adhered to. You will obviously provide first aid and care for any victims of accidents or injuries at the workplace. After injury or illness, it will also be your task to help the employee to cope with the return to work.

You will also have to deal with a variety of questions, give advice on personal problems and help the work force to keep in good health by promoting a healthy life style. Some of your patients may be suffering from stress and you will have to help them to deal with this. You will find plenty of variety if you choose this type of nursing.

Revising the points

● Identify health hazards.

● Support and care for employees.

NURSING IN A PRACTICE

Practice nurses are usually registered nurses who provide nursing care either in a health centre or within the practice of a general practitioner by whom they are employed. Many of them work part-time and, as the hours are flexible, it is a useful option for those with small children.

Taking a course

Although at the moment you do not need any further training to be a practice nurse, it is possible to do a ten day course at some colleges of nursing. There are also study days dealing with specific areas that would be helpful. You might attend courses on wound care, ear syringing and immunisation programmes. These would also be of use to you in fulfilling your PREP requirements.

Treating your patients

Much of your time in the surgery will be spent on routine tasks. You will be required to take blood tests, dress wounds, remove stitches, syringe ears and perform cervical smear tests. Many of the patients you will see regularly and this will enable you to build up a friendly relationship.

Part of your role will also be to advise travellers to foreign countries on health care and give the relevant vaccinations. Remember that a doctor must be present in the building when giving some of these in case the patient reacts to the vaccine; this rarely happens.

Promoting a healthy life style

You will also be responsible for encouraging healthy living. You will do health checks on the over 75s either in the surgery or in their own homes and also on those newly registered patients. You may also run a variety of specialised clinics in the following areas:

● asthma

● diabetes

● epilepsy

● hypertension

● weight control

● family planning (usually in conjunction with a doctor)

● well person.

Should you discover any problem that requires individual help, you should inform the GP. You may also find some of your clients could benefit from the services of a physiotherapist, occupational therapist, chiropodist or even a specialist nurse. If so, you should contact these professionals.

Negotiating your pay

Although your pay is likely to be comparable to that of your colleagues who are working for the NHS, you will negotiate it with your employer. You will also have to discuss arrangements for sickness benefit, holiday pay, maternity leave and pensions.

Revising the points

● Work in a health centre or for a GP.

● Carry out routine tasks.

● Promote a healthy life style.

● Run clinics.

GOING INTO SCHOOLS

If you have trained in adult or children's nursing, you could choose to become a school nurse. However, as in most other specialities, you will need to have several years' experience before applying for training in this field. The training is at diploma or degree level and you should apply to the appropriate college of nursing.

Meeting the children

As a school nurse you would take an active part in educating the pupils about important health issues and monitoring their progress.

You would be expected to carry out regular health checks. You would check the children's weight and height and carry out hearing and sight tests as well as giving routine vaccinations. You would probably be responsible for several schools and the pupils would be between the ages of three and 18.

You should be alert to any health problems and should inform the school medical officer of these. It is also your responsibility to advise and support parents whose children have any problems.

Dealing with special needs

Some of your pupils may have specific health problems and may need specialist help. You will have to store their medication safely and make sure that it is taken at the right time. Nowadays children with physical disabilities – sometimes wheelchair-bound – often receive education in mainstream schools. These may be receiving treatment from physiotherapists, occupational therapists, speech therapists or others. You will work closely with other professionals treating children in any of your schools. Any children who could benefit from extra help from other professionals must be referred to the appropriate department.

Revising the points

● Carry out health checks and give injections.

● Educate pupils about health issues.

● Liaise with other professionals.

NURSING IN THE PRISON SERVICE

The Prison Service employs about 1600 nursing staff. Most are registered nurses but some have NVQ qualifications in Care. The latter may have done courses in:

● acute care

● mental health and continuing care

● outpatient and clinic care.

Training as a health care officer

It is advisable to have had some experience after you have qualified before joining the prison service. Both general and psychiatric nurses are required. You may find that a community psychiatric nurse, who is not attached to the prison, will work with you on certain cases and this link with the community can promote a positive approach to mental health care within the prison.

Soon after you join the prison service, you will have a week's residential induction programme; this takes place at Newbold Revel Prison Service College in Rugby. Alternatively you may be able to attend the course daily at a Regional Centre near your own prison. Your travel expenses will be refunded. If you wish to become a health care officer, you will take the eleven week officer training course before specialising in health care. As a prison officer, you will have both a clinical and a custodial role.

Working in the prison

Much of the work you do will be similar to working in an outpatient clinic or as a practice nurse or occupational health nurse. You will have to deal with accidents and medical emergencies so previous experience in an Accident and Emergency department would be useful. There will be many instances of mental health problems so if you are a psychiatric nurse you may be in great demand to care for these patients. You will need skill in counselling and in running group therapy sessions.

Part of your work will be to promote good health; you may be expected to run clinics and prepare educational programmes to improve the health of your clients.

Combating drugs

Because the misuse of drugs and alcohol is so widespread in prisons today, you should be knowledgeable about the misuse of drugs and other substances and should know how sufferers can be treated. There are a number of English National Board (ENB) accredited courses related to drug and substance misuse and you are advised to take one if you wish to work for the prison service. Contact: The English National Board Careers Service, PO Box 2EN, London WIA 2EN. Tel: (0171) 391 6200 or (0171) 391 6205. You will need to know about:

● prevention

● detoxification

- long term treatment

- rehabilitation

- counselling

- education.

You may find that you become involved in a multi-disciplinary education programme to combat drugs within the prison and there may also be links with the community outside.

Finding a job

You will find advertisements for jobs in the national and local papers and in nursing journals. You could also write to the health care manager of the particular prison in which you are interested. For more information about nursing in the prison service, write to The Nursing Adviser, HM Prison Service Health Care, Cleland House, Page Street, London SW1P 4LN. You are likely to be paid on a D or E grade.

Revising the points

- Take a course in control and security.

- Train as a health care officer.

- Deal with emergencies.

- Counsel clients.

- Run clinics and educational programmes.

- Learn about drug misuse.

HELPING PSYCHIATRIC PATIENTS

You may decide to take the mental health branch of the Project 2000 course and train to be a mental health nurse. Instead of caring for people with physical problems, you will help those who principally have emotional and psychiatric problems. You will find the work very different from that of a general nurse. Your patients, also called clients, are referred to as psychiatric sufferers or clients with mental health problems.

Training to help psychiatric patients

During your training you will spend a great deal of time working on communication skills as you need to learn how to communicate with people who may be experiencing the world in a very different way from you. They may, perhaps, be convinced they are hearing voices or they may feel very depressed. You will learn how to deal with them through lectures, seminars, presentations, project work and role play. Your training will include a variety of placements where you will meet many people who have mental health problems. By the end of your training you will have experienced most aspects of psychiatric nursing.

Meeting the patients

You will meet patients with mental health problems as part of a community mental health team and in various settings:

● on a ward

● in a community home

● in a day centre

● in a private psychiatric hospital

● at a secure unit.

You may also work for a voluntary organisation specialising in a particular type of illness:

● National Schizophrenic Fellowship

● an organisation specialising in alcohol and drug rehabilitation.

Wherever you work, your clients will be suffering from paranoia, phobias, depression and/or addictions, often as a result of traumatic experiences. Your role is to help them live with their experiences so that their suffering may be lessened. Even a small improvement can be very rewarding for both of you.

Working as a community psychiatric nurse

A community psychiatric nurse (CPN) is one who works in the community, in a home or day hospital. You will need a great deal of experience before applying for this post. If you choose this option, you will form part of the community mental health care team.

Other members include a social worker, psychiatrist and clinical psychologist. Usually you will see clients at the team office but sometimes you may visit them in their homes. If you work in a community home, much of your work will involve helping your clients adjust to being back in the community. They may need help in the following areas:

● crossing the road

● applying for employment

● communicating

● learning work skills

● managing a budget.

If you work in a day hospital, you will do group work in the following areas:

● relaxation

● cognitive skills

● art and pottery (with the occupational therapy department)

● relative support.

Taking courses

Further training in this field will often be useful. Short courses are available at NHS Trust Hospital Training Departments. There may be courses on:

● managing aggression

● control and restraint

● communication skills.

The English National Board holds longer courses on:

● group dynamics

● behavioural approaches

● counselling.

To find out more about these contact the ENB. If you wish to stay in psychiatric nursing and gain promotion, you may find a degree in community mental health or psychology useful.

Advantages of working with psychiatric clients

● You have the opportunity to build up a relationship with people often discriminated against by society.

● It is rewarding to watch clients achieve life changes.

- You will discover more about yourself as you learn more about others.

- Frequently a uniform is not worn.

Disadvantages of working with psychiatric clients

- When you are new to the work, it may seem frightening.

- You do not make people physically better but try to help them cope with their problems.

- The work can be emotionally very exhausting.

- The patients may not be willing to receive your help.

Revising the points

- Your clients have psychiatric problems.

- Communication skills are essential.

- Clients are helped to adjust to going back to the community.

- Mental health nursing is very challenging.

- Helping the clients can be very rewarding.

WORKING AS A SALES REPRESENTATIVE

If you feel you would like to branch out from the healthcare service, working as a sales representative may appeal to you. You will find such positions advertised regularly in the nursing press. The work is very different from that of a nurse but the emphasis is still on customer satisfaction. You may take over from somebody who has already built up a list of customers or you may have to start from scratch and do this yourself.

If the latter, you will have to work hard at building a friendly and reliable relationship with the relevant people. You can offer to provide a teaching seminar on a subject which would enable you to promote your product. The key to success is to visit your clients regularly. There are many products which you could sell. Some are:

- patient lifting and bathing equipment

- wound care products

- intravenous (drip) therapy equipment

- specialist beds and mattresses
- continence products
- pressure area care products
- surgical equipment
- mobility aids
- pharmaceuticals.

As a sales representative you will usually enjoy several perks and although you will have a basic salary, commission is frequently offered too. You are likely to be provided with a company car and may also have access to a mobile phone, fax machine, home computer, private healthcare for yourself and family and an expenses allowance. In return you will have to meet sales targets, provide regular reports, attend meetings, travel long distances and meet deadlines.

Some of the skills you will require are:

- ambition
- commitment
- motivation
- energy
- determination
- confidence
- good communication and organisational skills.

Revising the points

- There are a variety of products you can sell.
- You may enjoy some perks.
- You must build up a friendly relationship with your clients.
- You must be prepared to work hard.

BECOMING A HEALTH VISITOR

There are not now so many opportunities for health visiting but this situation may change in the future. As a health visitor, you must be able to communicate well with people of all ages, particularly with the under fives and the elderly. You will find tremendous satisfaction in this demanding and challenging job which takes you into the community and into people's homes.

Training as a health visitor

To train as a health visitor you must be a registered general nurse with at least two years' experience. Training courses are at degree level and can be taken at some universities. You can do a full-time course lasting 51 weeks or a part-time one taking twice the time.

The course is extensive. Your role as a health visitor is to promote healthy living so you will study a variety of subjects to help you with the work in which you will be involved. Here are some of your study areas:

● care in the community

● the principles and practice of health visiting

● the sociology of health and illness

● child development

● how to help parents

● how to prevent illness and accidents

● legal and ethical issues in the community

● how to develop management skills.

Your course will consist of a mixture of theory and practical experience and you will be continually assessed. During the course you will be attached to a practising health visitor, who will help you to obtain the necessary experience and teach you the skills required. When you have completed your training, you are likely to be paid on a G grade but you can progress to higher grades as you become more experienced.

Assessing the community

It is advisable to remain in your first placement for at least two years so that you can gain relevant experience and get to know the people in your area.

It is essential that you make yourself aware of the needs of the community in which you are working. Are there elderly people living alone who would benefit from a visit from you? Do you have clients who have special needs? Have you identified any children at risk of abuse? Are there particular problems in the area which should be addressed?

It is your role to promote a healthy life style in your community by encouraging your clients to follow simple health guidelines. You also have a responsibility to identify any particular health hazards or accident 'black spots' and make the relevant authorities aware of them.

Helping mothers and children

You will visit new mothers after the birth and then at intervals until the child starts school. You will advise her on the care of the child and ensure that there are no health hazards or potential accident traps as her child grows. The midwife will also be involved both before and after the birth so it is important that you form a good relationship with this professional. Your primary concern is for the child's welfare. You may give advice about feeding the baby and weaning it. You will help the mother deal with problems associated with bringing up a child – crying, getting up at night and lack of sleep. As the child grows, you will encourage the mother to care appropriately for it, to seek dental care and to learn about health and safety. You will check the child's development and give the required immunisations.

If at any time you feel that a child is being ill treated or neglected, it is your responsibility to inform the G.P and Social Services and liaise with them about the best course of action.

Dealing with the elderly

You may have a high proportion of elderly people in your area. Some may live alone or with a spouse and some in nursing or residential homes. Some of them will have difficulty coming to terms with an illness or increased immobility and your role will be to provide support and help in whatever way is appropriate. In the case of the terminally ill, you will also have to help the family to cope with the situation and comfort the bereaved.

Organising support groups

One of your most interesting tasks will be to set up various support groups. These could include the following:

● new mothers

● smokers who want to give up

● parents of difficult teenagers

● relatives of the terminally ill or recently bereaved

- those who live alone and feel isolated

- women pregnant for the first time.

Liaising with other professionals
You might be located in a Health Centre or in a GP's surgery, although patients will be able to contact you without going through their GP. You will have the opportunity to work closely with the other professionals in the practice:

- midwives

- doctors

- district nurses

- social workers

.● practice nurses

Although you usually work alone, you are part of a community team and your colleagues will always be there to help you provide the service your patients need.

Giving talks
Occasionally you may feel it appropriate to promote health by giving talks on a particular subject. You might talk on any of the following:

- accident prevention

- parenting skills

- keeping healthy

- dealing with HIV/AIDS

- managing stress.

Counselling the needy
One of your primary roles will be to provide a listening ear and appropriate advice to those in need. One of your clients may have had sexual relations with a partner diagnosed as HIV positive. A teenage girl may be desperate because she's pregnant. Remember your role is to show compassion and provide help, not to be critical.

Finding career prospects
After you have worked for at least two years, you might choose to do some further specialist training in this field. This could provide the

opportunity for you to work as a field work teacher. You would teach and support health visitor students. You may wish to train to teach in a college of nursing or perhaps you would prefer to become a health visitor manager and lead a team.

Revising the points

● Promote healthy living.

● Be aware of the needs of your clients.

● Support the elderly.

● Organise support groups.

● Give talks.

● Counsel clients.

CASE STUDY

Lynne rises to the challenge of the baby clinic

Before taking the health visitor degree course, Lynne was a ward sister. She felt like a change and decided that working in the community would suit her. Although she had only been a health visitor for a few months she was asked to run the baby clinic on her own as no one else was available. She had done it before with a colleague and knew that unexpected problems could arise so she was a little nervous.

Her first 'patient' was a distraught mother whose four month old daughter had started crying at night and seemed constantly hungry. The mother told Lynne that the baby had a continuous cold and seemed hot. She also kept putting things in her mouth and rubbing her gums.

After asking a number of questions, Lynne suggested the child was probably teething and was also ready for solid feeding. The mother was told to give her child some baby rice for tea and to provide her with a water-filled teething ring toy which could be put in the fridge. The coolness would relieve the little girl's painful gums.

Lynne was glad she was able to reassure the mother there was nothing seriously wrong. For the rest of the morning, she dealt with easier cases. She was tired when the last patient had gone but she felt pleased with the way she had handled the clinic. She knew she was going to enjoy being a health visitor because she liked meeting a variety of people and was happy working either alone or as part of a team.

5

Working Abroad

If you feel you would like to work abroad for a time, there are *some* openings in various countries although not as many as there were a few years ago. You are advised to work in the UK for at least two years after you have qualified as few countries will take nurses with little experience. Some countries may require you to have specialist training in a particular field but this may be offered in the place of your choice.

As long as you continue to meet the PREP requirements while working abroad, your UKCC registration will continue. You will not therefore be required to undertake a Return to Practice Programme when you return home. However, don't forget that every three years you must do the equivalent of five days of study to maintain your professional development and registration.

ADAPTING TO THE COUNTRY

Whichever country you choose, it is essential that you do your homework before you go. Read as much as you can about the customs and culture of the country. If the language is not English, try to learn some before you go. You will find that even a little is appreciated by those you meet. If you wish to work in Europe, you are advised to learn the language of the country as you are unlikely to get a job without it.

Check on the weather you can expect. It may be considerably hotter than your native land so be prepared for this. Check on any inoculations you need and on general health care. In the developing countries you may have to take anti-malaria tablets.

By working overseas, you will learn flexibility and adaptability. You will discover there are several different ways to tackle a problem and you will have to adapt to conditions that may be very different from those in the UK. Ideas and developments in other countries influence and can enhance the British health care system so the experience and the expertise you will gain from working overseas will be invaluable.

GETTING ADVICE

The Royal College of Nursing has an overseas employment advisory service for members and you are advised to take advantage of this. It also keeps a register of members who live and work in other countries so could put you in touch with contacts in your chosen country. As a member of the International Council of Nurses (ICN) it could provide you with contacts in over a hundred countries. It will help you to plan overseas study visits and also aid you to find an appropriate placement.

The RCN also carries automatic world wide indemnity insurance cover for all its members.

ASCENDING THE CAREER LADDER

There is no right or wrong time for you to plan your work overseas. You may choose to go at the beginning of your career. In this case the experience you have gained will look well on your professional profile when you apply for promotion – although it does not guarantee a more senior post.

Perhaps you may prefer to reach the peak of your career and end it by working abroad when you will have so much to offer another country. You may choose to go for a number of years or for only a few months. A variety of options is open to you.

WORKING IN AUSTRALIA

If you wish to apply for a post in Australia, you must obtain a visa before you leave and you must register with the relevant State Nursing Board in Australia. Your rates of pay are likely to vary from state to state so check before you go.

Obtaining a visa

As you are unlikely to find *temporary* work as a qualified nurse, you are advised to apply for a migrant visa and this can take up to a year to obtain. The Australian Migration Branch has a 24 hour contact phone number: 0891 600 333.

Registering as a nurse

Before you are able to work as a nurse in Australia, you *must* have your UK qualifications checked by the Australian Nursing Council *and* apply for registration to the Registration Board of the area in which you hope to practise. You will have to pay a fee for both of these services. To have your qualifications checked, write to the Australian Nursing Council Inc, GPO Box 1907, Canberra, ACT 2601, Australia. The Australian High Commission will send you a list of the Nursing Registration Boards. The address is Australia House, Strand, London WC2B 4LA.

Finding a job

Australia House will also send you a list of the main public hospitals and you could write to them asking if they have any vacancies. Nursing posts are advertised in some Australian newspapers and magazines. Some of these are available at certain newsagents in this country. Write to Australia House for a list of the papers and magazines that include nursing advertisements. They will also send you a list of UK newsagents that sell these.

You may find yourself in an isolated post in the outback with only limited medical back up. In this case you will be responsible for the health of patients who live over a wide area. You may have to work alone with only a radio link to help you. You will learn a great deal and have to be very adaptable.

WORKING IN THE USA

There are now fewer openings for nurses in the United States as the federal government has introduced strict regulations about recruiting from overseas. However, there are still *some* openings for Registered General Nurses who have specialised in the adult branch of nursing.

Taking the CGFNS Test

Before taking up a post in the US, you may have to take an examination established in 1977 by the Commission on Graduates of Foreign Nursing Schools (CGFNS). The test, which is held twice a year and lasts a day, can be taken in the UK. It comprises English Comprehension and Nursing Proficiency. You will be expected to know something about the following branches of nursing: surgical, medical, paediatrics, obstetrics and mental health.

Not all states require you to take the test. Florida, California and Arkansas are three which do not.

You can obtain further information and an application form by writing to CGFNS, Fulbright House, 62 Doughty Street, London WC1N 2LS.

Finding a job

Before you can obtain a visa to work in the US, you must have a specific offer of employment. The International Department of the Royal College of Nursing can give you details of the US state nursing boards. You could then write to the appropriate board asking for a list of hospitals and job vacancies. Because of the vastness of the country, there is no national board of nursing so each state board produces its own regulations for the recruitment of overseas nurses. You must find out what the requirements are.

Obtaining a visa

When you have received the offer of employment, your prospective employer is responsible for applying for the visa you will require to work in the US. However, in order to process this, the state has first to satisfy itself that you have not been offered a post for which there is a qualified US nurse available. Once it has been established there is not and your labour certification has therefore been approved, the visa application can proceed. You would be wise to check the rates of pay as they vary considerably from state to state.

WORKING IN SAUDI ARABIA

Although there are fewer opportunities for UK nurses today in Saudi Arabia than previously, there are still more posts available than there are in other countries. The best way to find out about the nursing opportunities in that country is to write to the International Department of the Royal College of Nursing. You will also find advertisements in the *Nursing Times*.

Obtaining a permit

In order to work in Saudi Arabia you must have a valid work permit which will be obtained by your employer. Once you have started work, you will not be allowed to change your employment until your contract expires. When it does so, you may then apply for a different post and you will need a new work permit obtained by your new employer. You must carry your identification with you at all times. If you decide to terminate your contract early, you may have to reimburse your employer.

Adapting to a Muslim country

If you choose to work in Saudi Arabia, you must remember that you will experience a completely different culture from your own. The strict laws of the country are based on the Koran and you would do well not to fall foul of them.

Alcohol is banned and the authorities do not take kindly to foreigners who infringe their laws. Women are expected to dress modestly at all times. While you will not be expected to veil your face as many Saudi women do, you are advised to wear a long skirt and avoid short sleeves when in public.

Living in a compound

You are likely to be offered free accommodation. This will probably be a flat in a compound where other overseas staff also live. You may find that no charge is made for electricity and water. You will be provided with a phone and all national calls are free. However it is very expensive to phone home. Your rates of pay will probably be reasonable and you may be able to save up so that you can travel around the country.

Conditions are more relaxed in the compound and you will have the opportunity to use the communal swimming pool and take part in other leisure activities that are provided.

There will also be shopping facilities within the compound.

Nursing in a Saudi hospital

You are likely to find that your hospital, possibly managed by a British or American company, is a hi-tech, modern and well equipped complex but there will, of course, be a language barrier unless you speak Arabic. However, you will find that this is overcome as an interpreter is attached to every ward and department in the hospital.

WORKING IN THE DEVELOPING COUNTRIES

For most posts in the developing world you will require a minimum of two years' post registration experience, preferably with extra specialist training in midwifery or health visiting. You will usually be provided with free accommodation, which is likely to be very basic, and you will receive an allowance to cover your living expenses. Most posts will be offered through an international aid agency. Save the Children recruits experienced practitioners or you may become a VSO (Voluntary Service Overseas).

Some UK hospitals have links with hospitals in developing countries and if you are experienced, you may be able to visit one for a brief period of time to help the local practitioners develop their expertise.

Finding a job

To find out about working in developing countries write to the International Health Exchange, 8–10 Dryden Street, London WC2E 9NA. They produce a magazine, *The Health Exchange*, and this has a job supplement which advertises jobs from most of the international aid agencies like Save the Children Fund and Oxfam. Every month posts are advertised for health workers in Africa, Latin America, Asia and other needy areas. The IHE also runs useful short courses for those who hope to work overseas.

If you have two years' experience, you are also entitled to join the International Health Exchange's Register of Health Workers. This is beneficial as the IHE is regularly asked to suggest potential candidates for posts which come up at short notice. If you work for a voluntary organisation, your contract will usually be for one or two years and it will be necessary for you to resign from your job in the UK. While the experience you will gain overseas is invaluable, it may not necessarily help your chances of promotion when you return.

Coping with the differences

If you obtain a post in a developing country, you will be working closely with local colleagues and helping them to develop their skills so that they can promote health care in their countries.

You might work with community leaders, local nurses and doctors and other health workers. You might even find yourself liaising with engineers or agricultural specialists in an attempt to improve health care in the community. As you will be forming part of a team, you will need to hone your communications skills and be diplomatic in your dealings with government officials and those who work for the voluntary sector.

You will also need to be adaptable and able to work under pressure. Conditions will be very different from those in the UK. Don't expect to find modern technology and all the resources you are used to. You will have to 'make do' with what is available and you will find that your planning and problem solving skills are greatly increased. Remember also that your working conditions may sometimes be dangerous and stressful and subject to rapid change.

The work you will do is unlikely to be specialised so the broader your experience, the more helpful it will be. Here are some of the areas in which you may work:

● nutrition

● community health care

- infection control

- immunisation

- health management and finance

- the care of mothers and children

- family planning.

In some countries you may be working in a clinic in the country rather than in a hospital in the town.

Working with a relief agency

The number of disasters around the world seem to be increasing and relief workers now need a vast range of skills and experience. If you are a qualified nurse who has already had experience working overseas, you might be contacted at short notice and asked to fly to an emergency area. Your posting will usually be for three to six months and in most cases your salary will still be paid and, when the emergency is over, you should be able to return to your post in the UK.

WORKING WITHIN THE EUROPEAN UNION

If you are a British citizen, you can work in one of the member states of the European Union (EU) without a work permit. However, if you plan to stay longer than three months, you will need to approach the appropriate Embassy to apply for a resident's permit. Your UK qualifications will usually be recognised by member states. You should obtain a 'Certificate of Experience' as evidence of your qualifications and experience. This can be obtained from the Department of Trade and Industry at the European Division, Ashdown House, 6th Floor, 123 Victoria Street, London SW1E 6RB. You may have to pay a small fee.

You should have at least passed A level in the appropriate language if you wish to work in Europe.

Finding a job

You will find posts advertised in the major nursing journals. Job vacancies can also be found at Jobcentres. Ask for an overseas job search. Explain what type of post you require, what qualifications you have and where you wish to work. You can obtain more detailed information from one of the Employment Services' teams of Euroadvisers who are trained employment advisers. You can obtain a list of Euroadvisers by writing to the Deputy Chief Nursing and Healthcare

Employment Consultant and asking for a copy of the leaflet, *Thinking of Working in Europe?* The address is Broadacre House, Market Street (East), Newcastle-upon-Tyne NE1 6HQ.

Factsheets about living and working conditions in the EU are produced by The Overseas Placing Unit (OPU) and should be available at your local Jobcentre. Alternatively you can obtain them by writing to The Employment Service, Overseas Placing Unit, Rockingham House, 123 West Street, Sheffield S1 4ER. They may also be able to tell you about rates of pay which will vary.

The Royal College of Nursing also produces a quarterly newsletter *EuroForum*. If you are serious about working in Europe, this will give you information about developments both in the European Union and in the rest of Europe.

LOOKING AT OTHER OPTIONS

There are two other options which may give you the opportunity to see something of other countries but this is not guaranteed. You may choose to nurse in the Armed Forces or to work on a cruise ship.

Working in the Armed Forces

There are limited opportunities for undergoing your initial training in the Armed Forces but all three services recruit qualified nurses.

Choosing the army

The army nursing corps is the largest of the three services and is known as Queen Alexandra's Royal Army Nursing Corps, QARANC. You are unlikely to be recruited after the age of 38 and this upper age limit is likely to be lowered in the future.

If you are under 25, you may apply to train with QARANC which has a contract with the University of Portsmouth to provide nursing training. To apply you will need at least five GCSEs at Grade C including English Language and a science subject. If you are successful, you will then undergo a rigorous eleven week army recruitment training programme.

Choosing the navy

Because Queen Alexandra's Royal Naval Nursing Service, QARNNS, is not as large as the army corps, it only recruits a small number of nurses. You must be between 18 and 33 but the upper age limit is likely to be lowered. To train with QARNNS, five GCSEs are required but particular subjects are not stipulated.

Choosing the RAF

If you wish to apply for Princess Mary's Royal Air Force Nursing Service, PMRAFNS, you must be under 27. The entry requirements are the same as for the navy.

Finding employment in the service

If you are a registered nurse with several years' experience, you may be recruited into the service of your choice as an officer. If you are recently qualified, you may join as a non-commissioned staff nurse and seek promotion later. One advantage of doing your training in the service is that you are paid a salary while training and guaranteed a job once you are qualified. Find out the rates of pay from the appropriate recruiting centre.

Joining the reserves

All the services have reserve forces. If you would like to find out more about life in the Armed Forces, but do not yet want fully to commit yourself, you could serve in the reserves. This would prove an advantage if you were to apply for a commission later.

Nursing on a cruise ship

To work on a cruise ship, you should be a registered nurse with at least three years' experience of working on dry land before you attempt to sail the ocean! It would be an advantage if you have previously worked in an operating theatre, an accident and emergency department, an intensive care unit and in private medicine. Don't worry if you haven't experienced all of these. It is also helpful if you have taken an Advanced Life Support course. This is usually a two day course run by the training department of a hospital. Although there is no fixed age limit, a ship's nurse would normally be aged between 25 and 40.

Seeking the vacancies

To find the post you are searching for, write to the cruise line of your choice asking if they have an appropriate vacancy. You can find out the address from your local travel agent.

Dealing with your patients

Your duties would include dealing with minor ailments and injuries and also emergencies. There will be a doctor in charge of the medical centre and you will assist him when necessary. You may also have to carry out immunisations and administer first aid.

Enjoying your pay
Your salary is likely to be higher than that you would receive ashore and during the cruise you will have little opportunity to spend it so you should be able to save.

CHECKLIST

● Write to the appropriate authority for information.

● Learn as much as you can about the country.

● Try to learn the language if necessary.

● Be adaptable.

● Learn from your experiences and apply them to your work.

CASE STUDY

An eye-opening experience in Uganda

John, a health visitor, was delighted when he was invited to go as an adviser to a Ugandan hospital for two weeks. It would be his first visit to a developing country. He was to be accompanied by Susan, an experienced midwife, who had worked in Uganda previously.

Although he had been warned to expect the unexpected, John was not really prepared for what he discovered. He found the much slower pace of life in Uganda very frustrating.

'The only time the Africans go fast is when they're driving,' he said on his return. 'Then they exceed all speed limits.'

He was given very basic accommodation in a block of flats and was startled to find no hot water. The first night there was a power cut but fortunately he had been warned about this and was prepared with candles. The flats were isolated from the main hospital so he was grateful to know that a security guard slept nearby.

The first day he and Susan were taken on a tour of the hospital by the medical director and a senior nurse. John was taken aback by how spartan the wards were. Each contained about 20 iron beds ranged against the grey walls. Food was not provided by the hospital so the relatives, who were responsible for feeding the patients, slept on the bare floor beside the beds.

Both Susan and John were dismayed at the lack of facilities and medicines and found that one of their main roles was to listen attentively to the local medical staff explaining their difficulties. Although they had brought some supplies from the UK, these were a mere drop in the ocean compared with what was needed. They gave some lectures to the nurses but as these always started late, they were not sure whether they were beneficial. They made some suggestions for improving conditions and making the best use of the facilities available but they were frustrated by the little they could do.

However, they were impressed when they went out with the 'home care team'. This consisted of a nurse, a dispenser and a counsellor who travelled round the country visiting patients who were unable to get to the hospital. AIDS was prevalent in the area and the group counselled AIDS patients as well as educating the villagers in primary health care and HIV prevention. John and Susan were fascinated when they were invited to watch a spectacular African dance which had been adapted to promote AIDS awareness! They were told that a number of people from different villages had been trained as 'community workers' in HIV/AIDS care and it was hoped to continue with this project.

John found his first experience of life in a developing country a rewarding one. The people were friendly and the country beautiful but he was sad he could do so little to improve conditions in the hospital. He was relieved to return home and resolved to 'count his blessings' before he complained again about conditions in the UK!

6

Trying the Independent Sector

WORKING IN A HOSPICE

Dame Cicely Saunders opened the first hospice, St Christopher's, in 1967. As long ago as 1948 she had had a dream of creating a peaceful environment where the terminally ill could be given the best help and meet death surrounded by care and love.

Today, thanks to her vision, there are many hospices all over the country, staffed by caring nurses and volunteers. Most of them are registered charities relying on funding from charitable giving of all types. They are expensive to run and the growth of hospice shops staffed by volunteers has helped to raise considerable sums. Hospice care is always free to patients.

Contrary to popular belief, hospices are *not* depressing places where people go to die; they are cheerful, friendly, relaxing places where patients have their own rooms, can receive visitors at any time and can order special diets.

Children are occasionally admitted to hospices, but most terminally ill children will spend time in specialist units attached to hospitals. As their illness progresses, they usually return home to be with their families at the end. However, one or two hospices especially for children have now been opened.

Attending a hospice

Not all patients are terminally ill. Some go into a hospice for a short period of time – usually a week to ten days – to give some respite to their carers. Others are there for specific medical reasons – perhaps to control pain or alleviate symptoms of their illness – while some may require specialist care for a short while.

Visiting the day care unit

Some hospices provide a day care unit where not more than ten patients attend on a regular basis from one to three times a week. The sessions usually start about 9.30 and end about 16.00. Those who attend all suffer from life threatening diseases and they are offered the services of professional care workers.

The unit is run by a team headed by an experienced registered nurse who works closely with the physiotherapist and occupational therapist attached to the hospice. Other therapists will also visit on a regular basis and doctors are always available for consultation. The patients can receive both group therapy and individual help.

Outings, such as to the theatre or the seaside, are sometimes arranged and there is usually a chapel where services are held and where visitors and patients can go at any time.

Nursing in a hospice

If you plan to work in a hospice you should take the ENB course 931, Care of the Dying. Also very useful would be the Diploma in Palliative Care which is offered by most colleges of nursing and can lead to a degree. You might choose to do either or both of these courses before starting work or you may prefer to study while you are working. When you have gained more experience, you might like to apply for a sister's or matron's post. You will find you work with both nursing auxiliaries and those who have NVQ care training. There will also be a number of volunteers who run the reception desk and provide other services. You will discover that counsellors specialising in family counselling and bereavement counselling are attached to the hospice. Macmillan nurses may be employed full time or visit frequently. They also visit patients in their own homes. Nurses who work in a hospice are usually paid the same as their colleagues who work for the NHS.

Revising the points

- Hospices are caring places.

- They are not only for the terminally ill.

- There is often a day care unit.

- Rates of pay are the same as the NHS.

BEING A MACMILLAN NURSE

Macmillan Cancer Relief was set up as a charity in 1911 by Douglas Macmillan whose father had just died of cancer. Today it provides specialist nurses and doctors to care for cancer sufferers. It also funds buildings and provides a medical and nursing education programme and an education resources unit.

Helping cancer patients

If you wish to be a Macmillan nurse, you should be fully trained and will need to undergo some specialist training to help you deal with cancer patients. There are different types of cancer and you may choose to specialise in one of them. You may be a specialist in leukaemia, breast cancer or cancers that affect children.

Working as a Macmillan nurse

As a Macmillan nurse you may be based in the community. In this case you would visit your patients in their homes, offering psychological support and helping to alleviate pain and the symptoms of the disease. You will also be able to advise on treatment options. You will not only support the patient but you will be there to help the relatives too.

If you work in a hospital, you will usually support your patient from the time the cancer is first diagnosed. You will be there when he or she is having treatment and will be able to advise the relatives about their support.

Your services will be free to anyone suffering from cancer if they are being treated by the NHS. You will always work closely, both in the community and in the hospital, with other health care professionals. Your salary initially will be paid by the Macmillan Fund but, once your post is established, your salary will come from the local NHS trust for whom you work.

WORKING FOR AN AGENCY

If you like the idea of flexibility in time and place, you might consider working for a nursing agency. You could be employed on a full-time basis or you could supplement your income by working on your days off or during your holidays. Whichever you choose, you must inform the agency each week or month when you are available. They will then call you when they have work for you on those days. If you specify a particular place to work, this may limit the number of hours you are offered.

Looking at places of work

You may be offered work in a variety of venues:

● private hospital

- hospice

- NHS Trust hospital

- nursing home

- residential home

- day care unit

Coping with the stress

Unlike working full-time in one place of work, you may not know where you are working from day to day. This can be stressful as you are unlikely to receive any pay if you don't work. Your pay may be comparably higher than you would receive on the Whitley scale but remember that it is unlikely you will be paid if you have to take time off for illness or if you need a holiday. Your pay will, of course, depend on how many hours you work. If you have skills in intensive care, nursing sick children or other specialist skills, you will receive a higher rate of pay.

Appreciating the benefits

If you work full-time for a nursing agency, you may be offered a holiday and sick pay deal. You will be able to experience many types of nursing, meet new people and discover a variety of work places. You may find that you enjoy nursing in a particular area that you had not considered before.

Revising the points

- You can work full-time for an agency.

- You can work in your free time to supplement your income.

- You will experience a variety of work places and different areas of nursing.

- You have flexibility.

NURSING IN A BOARDING SCHOOL

If you enjoy working with young people, you might consider taking a position in an independent boarding school. Most of these are divided into houses over which a matron presides. She is not usually a qualified nurse. She is in *locto parentis* and her role is that of a house mother. Her responsibility is the welfare of the pupils. She organises their washing, does their mending, dispenses medicines, deals with minor ailments and provides a listening ear where necessary. She is usually on call for 24 hours a day. She will, of course, have free days when a colleague will cover for her. She will probably hold a morning surgery during which she will give out chits to any pupils who need to see the doctor or resident nursing staff.

Working in the sanatorium

A school that boards several hundred young people has to have resident nurses; these are usually a sister and a staff nurse who share the work between them. If you choose this option, you will be given a flat on the premises and your work base will be the sanatorium or health centre. This will contain a number of beds, treatment rooms and a room for counsellors as well as an office. Like the matron, you will be on call for 24 hours a day but will have time off. A doctor will probably hold a surgery every morning except Sunday and the school may also have regular visits from a physiotherapist and a school counsellor.

Using your experience

Your work will be very varied. You should be a registered nurse with some previous experience. Particularly useful would be work as a practice nurse or in an accident and emergency department. If you have worked with young people in any capacity, this also would be useful. There is no specific training for sanatorium nurses although the Royal College of Nursing occasionally runs relevant courses.

Appreciating the variety

Your day as a staff nurse or sister in a boarding school is unlikely to follow a routine pattern. It will be flexible because you never know what the day will bring.

Morning surgery

You will probably hold a surgery with the doctor every morning. You will see pupils who have been referred to you by the matron of their house. Your patients' ailments will not differ greatly from those seen by a nurse in general practice.

Some of your patients will have colds and store throats; others may have psychological problems. You may have to recognise the signs of drug abuse and know how to discourage it. You may have to take out stitches or give injections. If bed rest is required, it is likely you will refer the child back to the matron for ongoing care. The beds in the sanatorium will be used if there is an epidemic or if a sick child is unable to return home for the holidays.

Sports injuries
During the afternoon, you may have to deal with a number of sports injuries. Some will be minor and some more serious. You will have to decide if any injured child needs a doctor's care or should go to hospital.

Looking after the staff
You will also hold surgeries for both the teaching staff and the ancillary staff so you could be responsible for the health of nearly a thousand people. It is not a post for the faint hearted! Supporting the house matrons and other house staff and giving them advice on the care of their charges will also be your responsibility.

Dividing the terms
You will be expected to perform certain tasks each year and some of them are done at specific times. An ongoing requirement will be to teach life skills to the adolescents in your charge. You should explain how to prevent accidents and illness.

Christmas term
In September you will have to give all the new pupils a thorough medical examination. Their notes must be written up meticulously. You will be responsible for noting their height and weight and any medical problems they have. You will also do sight and hearing tests and give BCG vaccinations and boosters.

Spring term
During this term it is likely that you will be involved in health screening your 16 year old pupils. As well as the basic tests, this will include giving guidance on avoiding drug and alcohol abuse.

Summer term
The summer term will be taken up with a variety of holiday vaccinations and boosters. You may have to give advice to pupils who are travelling abroad for the first time as well as providing appropriate injections for experienced travellers whose parents live overseas.

Networking with colleagues
Working in a boarding school is often a lonely position and you will frequently have to act on your own initiative. You may have colleagues

in another school upon whom you can call in emergency but they may not be available when you need them. You may occasionally be called upon if there is an a nearby accident or situation that does not involve the school.

The Boarding Schools' Association runs some courses that may be of limited use to you. 'Issues in Boarding Education' will give you an overview of boarding school life and deals with problems you might encounter. More helpful would be 'Perspectives on Health and Development in Middle Childhood and Adolescence'.

The same association also has an annual conference for boarding school house staff and sanatorium sisters. This would be useful for any nurses who work in boarding schools. It would be an opportunity for you to network with other colleagues and discuss common problems. This can be included in your personal professional profile to keep up your PREP requirements.

To find out more contact the Boarding Schools' Association at Ysgol Nant, Valley Road, Llanfairfechan, Gwynedd, North Wales LL33 0ES. Tel: (01248) 680542.

Noting the skills

Any work you have already done with young people will be valuable experience for working in a boarding school. You will also need the following skills:

- flexibility

- ability to work on your own initiative

- a sense of humour

- stamina

- good communication skills.

Revising the points

- Previous experience in an A and E department or as a practice nurse would be useful.

- You are on call 24 hours a day.

- Your work will be varied and interesting.

- You must be flexible and able to work alone.

NURSING IN A PRIVATE HOSPITAL

If you would like to work in a private hospital, you will find the nursing is little different from that in an NHS Trust hospital. Most of the patients will be having consultations, health screening, operations and sometimes intensive care nursing in a special unit. You will work with other qualified nurses and health care assistants and are likely to be responsible for a group of patients. The clinics and wards will consist of nursing offices and private rooms for the patients.

To fulfil your PREP requirements you will be encouraged to attend study days and courses. These are likely to be funded or part funded by the hospital. You may have a positive performance review annually to check your professional development.

As private hospitals tend to be smaller than NHS ones, the opportunities for promotion or specialisation are more limited. However, higher grade nursing positions, like manager, training officer or standards and audit nurse do exist in some hospitals.

Your salary will be based on your experience and skills. It is usually in line with or slightly higher than the Whitley scale of pay. After about six months, you can expect to receive medical insurance including health screening for yourself and your dependants.

Revising the points

● Private patients have the same nursing needs as NHS patients.

● Promotional or specialist nursing posts may be limited.

● Professional development will be maintained.

CARING FOR THE ELDERLY

The elderly are an important section of our community and caring for them is a growing industry. As a nurse, you might find your niche working with senior citizens. There are plenty of openings.

Working in a residential or nursing home

Residential homes provide care for those who need help with some aspects of their daily lives. The residents appreciate the availability of professional help should they require it. In nursing homes most of the residents require greater nursing care as they can do little for themselves. All residential care homes are expected to provide 24 hour nursing care if they have over six residents. A number of homes are now dual registered; that means they provide residential *and* nursing care.

In most homes the residents have their own rooms; there is a communal dining room where meals are served to them but they may eat in their own rooms if they prefer. Occasionally residents share rooms and facilities are usually available for married couples. There is a lounge where they can relax and where entertainment is provided.

Residents in either type of home may include elderly people who are normally cared for at home but whose carers need a break. They will stay for a short while and this is known as 'respite care'. Some elderly people you will care for may be convalescing after a major illness or operation. Your role will be to care for them until they are able to return home.

Some homes are run by the local authority, some are run privately and others are managed by the voluntary sector. Charities like the Church Army, connected to the Anglican Church, run a number of homes for senior citizens who can no longer live at home. They aim to cater for 'the physical, emotional, social and spiritual needs' of all their clients. The Methodist Church also runs homes. Some establishments have the luxury of a four star hotel; others may not have the same standard of luxury but a high standard of care is still provided.

In homes which are members of a group the salary scales are usually fixed, as it is in some church homes. In smaller independent establishments you may have to negotiate your salary.

Obtaining specialist training

The English National Board (ENB) introduced new post-registration professional and academic awards in 1992. Colleges of nursing and universities offer these courses to enable you to improve your skill and increase your expertise when working with the elderly. Training in rehabilitation nursing and other areas related to elderly people will improve the quality of care you offer them.

Age Concern also offers a number of courses which would be helpful if you are working with the elderly. There are courses on helping those suffering from depression and dementia as well as others which would help you deal with any emergency conditions you might encounter. How would you cope with a stroke victim, someone suffering from hypothermia, cardiac arrest or epilepsy? There are also courses which aim to improve your management skills. These would be helpful if you are interested in becoming the manager of a home. Among the skills covered are self management, staff management and communication skills.

Making the most of your career opportunities

Career opportunities are expanding in this field. You could work as a staff nurse, sister or manager. You could even eventually become manager of a group of homes; or perhaps you might choose to lecture and lead seminars in this field, thus providing continuing education for other nurses.

If you choose to work with elderly people, you will find the magazine *Caring Today* helpful.

Revising the points

● There are both nursing and residential homes.

● They are run by voluntary organisations or the private sector and social services.

● Take a course run by the ENB.

● Read the magazine *Caring Today*.

CASE STUDY

A day in the life of a nursing home matron

Beth is an experienced registered nurse who is the matron of a nursing home. She has done a number of training courses to help her with her work; these include courses on creative activities, dementia, first aid and focus on spirituality.

Beth's diary

After I'd received the report from the night staff, I went round to check on all the residents. When I went into Edith's room, she flung the covers off her bed to show me she was dressed! She had her pants on her head and she'd pulled her tights over her slippers! She gets more confused every day. The smell as I opened Mabel's door nearly knocked me back. She was plastered all over with faeces. The poor soul is incontinent and faecal smearing is a well-known side effect of dementia. Putting my hand over my nose, I staggered to the window to open it.

It took me and Jane, one of the care assistants, ages to clean her up. Then we had to strip some of the residents' beds and wash or bath them. I took the dirty linen down. Some of it had to be soaked to sanitise it before I could put it in the washing machine.

The phone went as I was taking Doris to the toilet so I called Jane and rushed into the office. I wish I had a secretary. The phone never stops ringing. It was nearly nine by the time all the residents were sitting down to breakfast. Most of them need help with their food. Two of the care staff were serving them. Emily tipped pepper all over her porridge and Doris put her coffee cup in the middle of the table and was busy stirring her saucer with a spoon! I went round dispensing drugs and signing the patients' charts as I gave them their medicine. I was just in time to stop Jack, who's diabetic, eating a whole jar of marmalade!

After breakfast I assigned the staff their jobs and we shepherded the residents to the lounge where someone was coming in to do an entertainment for them. Jane and I continued tidying the bedrooms and washing linen until we could collapse with a brief cup of coffee. Some visitors arrived before I'd finished, so I had to show them round. Then I had to put a new dressing on Emily's leg and give Jack his injection before going to the office to catch up on some paperwork. The doctor came just as I sat down so I had to take him to see Jack.

I gave out the second dosage of medicine at lunch time and afterwards I spent some time with Edith, who is now bedridden and needs to be turned frequently. After that, I managed to fit in a brief staff meeting. We always have to have at least three staff on duty. The ratio has to be eight patients to one member of staff. In the middle of the meeting, Emily fell over in the lounge and cut her head on the corner of the mantelpiece. There was blood everywhere. Jane dialled 999 while I mopped her up and rendered first aid. Any head injury has to go to hospital.

The ambulance arrived very promptly and I sent Jane with the patient. I don't think she's badly hurt — just shaken. By the time they'd taken her off, it was almost 15.30 — the official end of my shift!

I still had a mound of paperwork to do so I sat down in the office hoping there'd be no more emergencies before I left. Brian, my replacement, arrived so I gave him my report and retired to my room for a much needed cup of tea before settling down to do the work I hadn't had time to do during the day.

7

Choosing to Be a Midwife

If you choose to be a midwife, you will have wonderful experiences as you will be involved with the birth of a new baby and all the joy that goes with it. At times it will also be a challenging and sad job. You will have to look after very sick pregnant women and deal with the birth of deformed or dead babies. You will be trained to cope with these traumatic situations. However, your role as a midwife involves more than delivering babies. You are a professional who is responsible for helping a woman to maintain good health while pregnant and for caring for her and her new baby for at least 28 days after the delivery.

TRAINING AS A MIDWIFE

You do not have to complete general nursing training before taking up midwifery training. At 18 or as a mature student you can have direct entry to a midwifery course. The training is a full time three year diploma course taken at a university. It is likely to become a degree course. The minimum entry requirements are:

● five GCSEs – Grade C or above including English language, maths and a science

● evidence of recent relevant work experience.

If you do not have these, the following qualifications may be acceptable:

● GNVQ advanced level

● SVQ at level three including English and a science

● BTEC higher national certificate or diploma.

There may be other acceptable qualifications. Contact the university to find out. If you are a qualified nurse, then a shortened 18 month diploma course is available. When sending your registration entry requirements, enclose the names of two referees and evidence of recent study.

The course consists of semesters which are broken down into academic blocks; these are completed at the university and at practical placements. To complete these, you will have to travel to more than one hospital in the region. The areas you visit will include:

- antenatal clinics and wards

- post-natal clinics and wards

- delivery suites

- neonatal intensive care units

- the community.

You will have practical supervised experience to equip you to work as a competent midwife.

ACQUIRING EXPERIENCE

As a newly qualified midwife, you may be given a contract by a hospital trust; you will work in different departments in the hospital. You can consolidate your training and have access to supervision if you need it. Your experiences will be varied and will include:

- monitoring pregnant women (taking blood pressure, urine tests and scans)

- delivering a baby

- assisting with a venteuse or forceps delivery

- preparing a woman and her partner for a caesarean section

- checking the health and development of a new born baby

- administering vitamins and medicines to the new baby

- teaching new parents how to bath their babies

- advising mothers about feeding their babies

- assisting an experienced midwife to care for a premature baby nursed in neonatal intensive care.

GAINING SKILLS

To practise as a midwife you must inform your supervisor (manager) that you intend to practise each year. You will be responsible for the effective care of the woman and her baby until a month after the birth. You will be helped to develop the following essential skills:

- communicating effectively
- deciding on priorities
- counselling
- teaching
- flexibility
- coping with emergencies
- reading and applying research
- self-management.

You are not expected to be an expert and you will be regularly appraised by your supervisor who will help you to identify which skills need developing and how this may be achieved.

LOOKING AT JOB POSSIBILITIES

As you gain experience as a midwife, you may decide to remain in hospital work – on wards, in clinics or in a delivery suite. Alternative positions are now becoming available. Some hospital trusts are employing advanced midwife practitioners. Training, for these midwives, involves learning about specific techniques taught by the trust to aid development and reduce the workload of other members of the team. Another position is that of a scanning midwife. As an expert on performing and reporting on scans, you can reassure expectant mothers or detect potential problems. There are also job possibilities in the following areas:

- HIV and AIDS
- drug dependency
- research and practice development
- standards and audit
- management and teaching.

WORKING IN THE COMMUNITY

Perhaps you may choose to work in the community. You may be based at a health centre or in a GP's surgery. You will monitor the development of the pregnancy in the woman's home and at your clinic. If there is any cause for concern, you must arrange for a specialist doctor to see the woman. During the pregnancy, you will offer parentcraft (ante natal) classes where parents learn about some of the experiences they might have and what choices they can make.

Your role as a midwife will vary according to the area in which you work. In some areas you will be involved with the delivery of the baby while in others the hospital midwives will be responsible for this. You must give the new mother plenty of encouragement, advice and support in all these areas:

- birthing positions

- pain control options

- feeding

- baby hygiene

- post-natal exercises

- sleep deprivation

- handling emotions.

You must also monitor the healing of the mother and the development of the baby until their care is handed over to the health visitor.

TAKING FURTHER TRAINING

If you wish to specialise in a particular area of midwifery or want promotion, you may need to undergo further training. The English National Board provide both long and short courses. Write to them for a list of the courses on offer. If you wish to work in neonatal intensive care, an appropriate course would be beneficial. If you prefer to work in the community, you will find the family planning course useful. Other courses available include working with drug dependants and with HIV and AIDS sufferers. The midwifery training department in the university also provides further training on various topics like foetal heart monitoring and the use of anaesthesia.

CHECKLIST

● A variety of work is on offer.

● You can specialise.

● Work in the community provides variety.

● Keep up your training.

CASE STUDY

Sandra has been a community midwife for fifteen years. She thoroughly enjoys her work which involves making sure pregnant women remain well and their babies develop as expected. Today she is going to be busy as yesterday afternoon three new mothers and their babies returned home from hospital.

Before visiting them, Sandra, and the student midwife working with her, took a parentcraft class where they discussed pain control methods with the expectant mothers; Sandra was delighted there were a number of husbands present. It was usually a well-attended session. Because there were lots of questions, it ran over the allotted time.

However, before lunch, Sandra had time to make a home visit to one of the new mothers and her baby. She checked the baby's weight, skin and eye condition and asked if there were any feeding problems especially as the mother was breast feeding. She was told the mother's breasts were very sore. Sandra recommended an ointment that could be used to soothe and suggested that nipple shields might be worn. She also helped the mother to position the baby in a more appropriate way when feeding.

She has great sympathy with the mothers as she remembers her own experience. Although her children are now teenagers, she finds that many of the problems she experienced when they were babies help her to emphathise with the new mothers and to offer appropriate advice and encouragement.

After lunch, Sandra makes her two other home visits and then returns to her office to catch up on some paperwork.

8

Working as a Nursery Nurse

If you wish to work with children who are well and have the choice of a variety of settings, nursery nursing may be right for you. To find out more write to the following addresses: The National Nursery Examination Board, 8 Chequer Street, St Albans, Hertfordshire AL1 3XZ and The Association of Nursery Training Colleges, The Princess Christian College, 26 Wilbraham Road, Fallowfield, Manchester M14 6JX.

TRAINING TO BE A NURSERY NURSE

The National Nursing Examination Board Diploma is the most widely recognised course. The other one is the BTEC National Diploma in childhood studies. Each of these allows you to work as a qualified nursery nurse. The courses can be taken at colleges of further education or at private colleges.

Studying for the NNEB diploma

To apply for the NNEB diploma you will require three GCSEs or an intermediate level GNVQ in Health and Social Care; however, if you are a mature applicant, these are not necessary. If you wish to study full time, it will take you two years to complete the diploma but it can be taken as a part time course over a longer period of time. The latter gives mature students with family commitments more flexibility in their studying. The following subjects will be studied through a variety of learning methods:

- health

- social studies

- art

- music

- nutrition

- education
- computing.

As part of the course you will work in a variety of settings.

Taking the BTEC course

The BTEC course lasts for two years full-time. To apply you will need four GCSEs or an intermediate GNVQ unless you are a mature student in which case these are waived. Your studies will include sociology, psychology, art and craft. Practical placements also form part of your work and you will be expected to deliver presentations to your fellow students.

Providing a character reference

In addition to your academic entry requirements, you must also provide the name of a referee who can vouch for your character. In order to offer you a place on a childcare course, the college needs to be reassured that you are a responsible person who, in the future, can be relied upon to take proper care of the children who are entrusted to you.

WORKING IN A HOSPITAL

If, when qualified, you choose to work in a hospital, you will be expected to work shifts which will usually include weekends and bank holidays. You are likely to work on a children's ward helping the children's nurses to nurse the child back to health. Alternatively you could train to work as a hospital play specialist on the children's ward as play is an important part of the child's rehabilitation.

You might also work in a maternity department supporting the midwives and helping the new mothers to learn how to care for their babies; you may teach them how to bath their offspring, how to care for the child's eyes and umbilical cord and you might also give advice on feeding.

A neonatal intensive care unit may make use of your services. Here you would help the midwives care for the baby and support and encourage the mother.

WORKING IN A NURSERY

There are different types of nurseries but the nature of the work is very similar. You might work in:

- a social services nursery

- a private nursery

- a hospital nursery

- a local education authority nursery school.

The age of the children will vary as some nurseries take children from as young as six weeks while others prefer them to be six months old. If you are looking after babies, your work revolves around their needs. You will feed, change, stimulate and cuddle them. As the children grow older, you will aim to aid their physical, emotional, social and mental development in a variety of ways. Some of these are:

- arranging team games to teach them social skills

- providing puzzles and books for mental stimulation

- physical activities could include: playing with sand and water, painting and drawing, or going for walks.

Older children, who need to be prepared for school, have to learn the following skills:

- putting on their coats

- putting on their shoes

- learning manners at meal times

- going to the toilet and washing their hands.

They will also be involved in National Curriculum Key Stage One work like counting and learning the alphabet. Look in your local bookshop for Key Stage One material or ask for help from your library. You will normally work office type hours to accommodate the parents whose children you are minding. However, some parents may work longer hours or be on shift work so you may be asked to adjust your hours and even work at weekends.

BEING A NANNY

When you are employed by a family, you will usually be looking after one, two or sometimes more children during the day while the parents are at work. You may live with the family but have your own room and bathroom; it is likely you will eat with the family. If you live in, you will earn less as your food and accommodation is provided. Alternatively, you could travel to work each day. This may require a very early start if the parents leave for work early in the morning.

Advantages of working as a nanny

● You are provided with accommodation, meals and possibly a car.

● You may have free time during the day while the children are at school.

● You will have freedom to decide what to do with the children.

● You can earn extra money by baby-sitting during your free time.

● You will have the opportunity to become friendly with other nannies.

Disadvantages of working as a nanny

● You may have to work long hours.

● You may be lonely.

● What you teach the children may not be reinforced by the parents.

● You may be exploited and expected to do housework.

● Extra baby-sitting may be required.

FINDING FURTHER OPPORTUNITIES

Working as a nursery nurse could be viewed as a job which lacks opportunity as you look after other people's children. However, a variety of opportunities is available to you if you wish to progress in the field. Working abroad is one option. The English nanny is still seen as the most acceptable in the world. This option could provide you with a high salary.

After you have had experience of working in a nursery, you could manage one or if you have the financial means you could even set up one of your own. There are courses available which provide specific information about this. Find out the regulations that apply before you decide on this option. There are laws relating to the number of adults required for a specific number of children and you will also have to check the health and safety aspects of the job.

You may decide you would like to teach. By gaining a teaching qualification, you would be able to teach others to become nursery nurses. Whatever you decide to do, you will find nursery nursing a rewarding job.

CHECKLIST

- You can gain a NNEB diploma or a BTEC national diploma.

- You can work in a hospital, a nursery or as a nanny.

- Career opportunities include working abroad and managing or owning a nursery.

- You will have a rewarding job.

CASE STUDY

Life *in loco parentis*

Sue is a nanny. She has charge of two children, a boy of two and a girl of five.

Sue's diary

Today has been really stressful. I can't wait until September when Charlotte goes to school. She is certainly ready for it. She constantly needs my attention to do things with her. This is very difficult when little Johnny is pulling everything out of the cupboards and trying to push small objects into his nose and ears.

I was trying to persuade him to shut the cupboard door when I was distracted by Charlotte climbing on to my back and feeling all over my head with her small fingers. When I asked what she was doing, she informed me she was looking for the eyes in the back of my head! I wish I did have some! I need them!

Because I'd taken my eye off him, Johnny managed to put a crayon right up his left nostril. It was safer not to touch it as I thought I would probably push it in further so I had to take him to hospital. Lorraine, his mother, didn't appreciate having to leave work and rush over. However, fortunately, she reassured me that it wasn't my fault and 'could have happened to anyone'. She told me she was very glad I was looking after the children because she trusted me and didn't have to worry about them.

They are a lovely family but looking after Charlotte and Johnny all day is exhausting,. Perhaps I should consider living out.

9

Becoming Self-Employed

After working in the NHS or private sector, you may decide that the way forward for you is self-employment. If you have been made redundant, are retired, returning to nursing or want a fresh challenge, you might consider this. Running your own business provides an exciting opportunity for you to use your experience, knowledge and skills to maximum effect without the restraints of being employed. However, think carefully before taking the plunge. The Royal College of Nursing produces a useful leaflet entitled *'Turning Initiative into Independence': Information for Would-be Nurse Entrepreneurs*. Write for a copy.

DECIDING TO WORK FOR YOURSELF

Make sure you have the right attributes to succeed. Evaluate yourself and decide on your area of interest. You must:

● be willing to take risks

● be enthusiastic

● be committed

● believe in yourself

● have self-confidence

● possess a desire to succeed

● be 'customer' oriented.

Using self-analysis

A self-analysis form would give you an idea where your strengths and weaknesses lie. You could consult a professional career consultant and pay for an analysis which should:

● assess your personality

● identify your constraints

- decide on your commitments

- find your reasons for change.

Assessing your personality
Are you competitive, cheerful, adaptable, anxious, shy, aggressive, sociable, reliable, hard working, gregarious, modest, well-organised?

Identifying your constraints

- Do you have family commitments?

- What is your financial position?

- Can you work flexible hours?

- Are you free to travel long distances and stay away from home for a period of time?

Deciding on your commitment
Are you willing to commit time and money in an effort to make your business succeed?

Finding reasons for change

- Do you have valid reasons for changing your lifestyle?

- Do you need the stimulation of a new challenge?

- Have you a burning desire to pioneer your ideas?

- Will you enjoy being your own boss?

- Do you crave independence?

- Will the financial rewards be greater than in your present job?

- Does working flexible and more congenial hours appeal to you?

Doing your homework

Speak to people who are already self-employed and find out about the positive and negative aspects. There are many books on the subject to help you discover whether this is right for you. Other sources of help include your local Trading and Enterprise Council, the local Chamber of Commerce and local Business Link Clubs. Doing your homework thoroughly will mean fewer pitfalls later on.

Questions to ask yourself

- What type of business?
- Who are your clients?
- How will you meet their needs?
- Will you employ others?
- What are your short and long term aims?
- How will you measure your success?
- How will you cope if you fail?
- Where will you find your capital?
- What hours will you work?
- What other commitments must you take into account?
- How will you market the business?
- Who are your competitors?
- Where will you provide your service?
- What will you charge?
- What insurance do you need?
- Who will keep your books?
- What about your pension?
- What equipment will you need?
- How much capital is required?
- Do you need access to the Internet?
- Is there a demand for your services?

SORTING OUT YOUR FINANCE

Before you set up your business, it would be useful to discuss your proposal with an accountant. He or she will help you to sort out your income tax, VAT, cash flow and advise you on all financial matters. Check the fee you will have to pay. Accountants are not cheap. Ask your colleagues if they can recommend someone.

Dealing with National Insurance contributions

When you are about to start your business, you must notify your local Department of Social Security office. As a self-employed individual, you will have to pay the flat rate of Class 2 National Insurance contributions. You will be asked to fill in the appropriate form CWF1. This can be found in leaflet CWL1 or can be obtained from the Social Security office. You can pay your contributions in two ways:

- by monthly direct debit

- by receiving quarterly bills issued in January, April, July and October. These can be paid at any bank, by GIRO or at a post office.

For further information contact: Contributions Agency, Class 2 Group, DSS, Newcastle upon Tyne NE98 1YX.

Dealing with tax

You will be sent a self-employment tax return which should be returned in April but your financial year will start on the day you start your business. You will pay tax *only* on the **profit** you make from your business. It is important that you keep detailed records of all expenditure and all your income. Keep all your receipts in case the Inland Revenue wish to inspect your books. Your profit or loss will be the difference between your expenditure and your earnings. A loss can be carried over to the following year. If your income is small, it may be worth doing your accounts yourself but if you want to avoid the hassle, an accountant can take care of everything for you, although you will have to provide detailed information. Remember that accountants' fees are quite high although these will count as expenses for tax purposes.

Dealing with insurance

If you have employees, you must take out employer's liability insurance in case they are ill or injured as a result of working for you. You should also have:

- professional indemnity (if you are a member of the RCN, you will already be covered for this)

- insurance to cover loss of earnings in case of illness or accident

- insurance against theft

- insurance against fire or damage to your premises.

Taking out a pension

You are recommended to take professional advice about private pensions. If you are a member of the RCN, you are entitled to independent financial advice. It is unlikely you will be able to continue with your NHS pension so you need to be aware of all the options open to you.

STARTING UP YOUR BUSINESS

Before you start, it is essential to produce a detailed business plan. You need to consider:

- your goals

- purchasing equipment

- renting premises

- taking on employees

- other expenses

- potential earnings

- potential profit.

Having taken the above into account, decide how much capital you need to start your business.

Raising the money

Decide how much capital you have of your own and how much you need to borrow. Whoever lends you the money will need to see your business proposal to satisfy themselves that you have a viable proposition. Ask the RCN for guidance on possible borrowers. You could approach a bank, companies, foundations or even private individuals.

Deciding on your fees

Once you have acquired the money, bought premises and set yourself up, you have to think about the fees you will charge. This will usually require negotiation between you and your client and it will depend upon what service you are offering. When deciding on a fee, it is essential to take into consideration your expenses. These can include:

- stationery

- computer

- telephone, fax machine, Internet

- running costs for equipment

- photocopying

- secretarial costs

- rent for your premises

- heat and lighting

- travelling time and petrol

- advertising.

Remember that all the above will count as expenses on your tax form and you will not have to pay tax on them. Other things to take into consideration when deciding on your fees are:

- what your competitors charge

- how much demand there is for your service

- the range of work and the level of expertise you offer

- the future demand for your services

- your expenses.

Invoicing your client
Before you undertake any work, agree with your client, in writing, the fee and conditions of your service. Buy an invoice book so you will have a record of what you have charged. Will you be paid at an hourly, daily, sessional or fixed rate? The service you offer will determine which method is most appropriate. You may, for example, offer a consultancy service and advise about setting up an out-of-hours call-out programme for district nurses. A fixed rate or daily rate may be more suitable than an hourly charge. If you do opt for a fixed rate, remember to estimate realistically the time required.

Remember that the frequency with which you invoice your clients will directly affect your cash flow. You can be paid weekly, monthly or immediately you have provided the service. If the bill has not been paid within a month, you are entitled to send a reminder. As this will take time, plan for it in your schedule.

SETTING UP A NURSING AGENCY

If there is sufficient demand for private nurses in your area, setting up a nursing agency could be a viable business proposition. To operate, you must obtain a licence from the local authority. They will provide you with information about regulations and inspections. If you decide on this route, the *RCN Guide for Good Practice in Nursing and Care Agencies* is essential reading.

OFFERING COMPLEMENTARY THERAPIES

As a qualified nurse, you may have taken further study in the field of complementary therapy. In hospital you would have used this to enhance your nursing care. As a self-employed complementary therapist, you can concentrate on providing this therapy as a total care and not part of that provided by an organisation. As you build up your client list, you will notice some patients frequently return for treatment. Someone who has a neck injury as a result of a car crash may benefit from periodic sessions from you to keep the problem under control. Before offering your complementary therapy service, choose the area in which you are interested.

- massage

- homeopathy

- reflexology

- aromatherapy

- hypnosis

- therapeutic touch

- acupuncture

- herbalism

- nutritional therapies

- art therapy

- shiatsu.

You are advised to take a comprehensive course on the subject you choose including supervised practice.

BECOMING AN EXPERT WITNESS

If you have expertise in a particular nursing field, you could act as an expert nurse witness. Your role would be to provide a written report and/or give evidence in court for a lawyer in cases of medical-legal litigation or personal injury claims. Information on training courses in this field is available from the Royal College of Nursing. With a little experience, this area of work could be financially rewarding.

OWNING OR MANAGING A RESIDENTIAL OR NURSING HOME

If you wish to care for the elderly, you might consider running a residential or nursing home. Before taking this step, you must study the guidelines and regulations. Approach the Social Services and the Health and Safety Executive first. Training your nursing staff and maintaining their PREP requirements is an important consideration. For further advice contact the Royal College of Nursing Forum for Nurses Working with Older People. See Chapter 6 for more details.

WORKING AS AN INDEPENDENT NURSE CONSULTANT

If you decide to become a nurse consultant, you will need experience and expert knowledge in your chosen field. Opportunities for work exist in:

- primary heath care
- specialist nursing
- research
- education
- management
- industry.

If you were to work in specialist nursing, you may offer advice or provide a complete service in an area like continence or infection control. You may advise other nurses or an organisation on setting up and running a project. Alternatively, you may have the opportunity to teach qualified nurses who are working in residential or nursing homes. You might also advise on the management of a home. As you will have had experience of working within the healthcare service, you will know where opportunities exist and which openings will suit you best.

TAKING UP COUNSELLING

Although it is advisable to have completed training in the skills of counselling before you promote yourself as a counsellor, this is not a statutory requirement. Numerous courses are available. These range from introductory, foundation and certificate level to diploma and higher degree level. The British Association for Counselling (BAC) provides courses and also recognises other courses that meet set criteria. You are advised to take training recognised by BAC. The address is British Association for Counselling, 1 Regent Place, Rugby CV21 2PJ. As a counsellor, you can work full or part-time in a variety of settings:

- youth services

- private practice

- voluntary organisations (*eg* Relate, Cruse, Mind)

- general practice

- churches

- specialist services (*eg* HIV/AIDS, drug and alcohol abuse)

- schools

- health service

- hospices.

CHECKLIST

- Do your homework thoroughly.

- Plan meticulously.

- Speak to other self-employed nurses.

- Look at all the options.

- Be aware of regulations and guidelines.

- Check there is a demand for your service.

● Acquire training in your field.

● Contact the RCN for help, advice and support.

CASE STUDY

Setting up as a counsellor

Janice is a qualified nurse who has worked for the NHS for a number of years. Among other courses she had taken a professional counselling course which had interested her greatly. She found she was able to do some counselling in her everyday job and knew it was something at which she excelled. She was sympathetic and always ready to listen.

For some time she had toyed with the idea of setting up as an independent counsellor as she already saw a few private patients in her spare time. One day in the canteen, Patricia, a physiotherapist, was talking about the clinic where she worked.

'It's an alternative therapy clinic,' she explained. 'There's a herbalist, an aromatherapist, a homeopath, a masseur and me. We have a spare room and are hoping to let it to a counsellor because we thought that service would fit in with the rest of us. You don't know anyone who might be interested, do you?'

That was the chance Janice had been waiting for. The premises were available, her services were required and she was sure it was the right move. She had already built up a client list and that would certainly expand if she worked in the clinic. That evening she prepared a business proposal and worked out how much she would need to borrow to set up her business. She was delighted it was less than she had expected.

She made an appointment to see her bank manager and showed him her figures. She waited in trepidation while he inspected them. But all was well. He agreed to lend her the money. The next few days were hectic as she was still working at the hospital. She had asked if she could work fewer hours and to her relief this had been agreed. So she had two days a week to concentrate on offering her counselling service and the hospital was happy to send new patients her way.

Her first appointment in her new clinic was a very sad one. Several weeks previously a young woman had been killed in a bad car crash and her husband and ten year old daughter were finding it almost impossible to cope with their loss. Janice listened and comforted them and as they left, she felt she had helped them a little. But she knew it would be many months before any signs of recovery would be shown. She had arranged to see them once a week for the time being.

She put the money the man had given her into her cash box and locked it. He had insisted on paying immediately and had not wanted an invoice but she had made one out and receipted it. It was her first payment in her independent venture. She wondered how long it would be before she would be able to pay back her loan and make a profit.

10

Returning to Nursing

It is now easier for nurses to return to work after a break than it was previously. Currently you do not *have* to take a refresher course but this will change in the year 2000 when a course is likely to become compulsory.

TAKING A BREAK

If you have nursed for less than 100 days (750 hours) during the past five years, this constitutes a 'break in practice'. From 1 April 2000, if you wish to return to nursing, you must complete a National Board approved Return to Practice Programme before you can renew your registration.

The United Kingdom Central Council for Nursing Midwifery and Health Visiting (UKCC) has produced specific standards relating to this and these are now part of the Council's policy for maintaining registration.

RETURNING TO PRACTICE

Return to Practice Programmes are already being offered by many colleges of nursing and these are available before the year 2000. If you think you would benefit from taking one, write to the appropriate college or the National Board for details.

Most courses usually last for 15 days to 20 days and their aim is to give you confidence to return to nursing as a competent practitioner. However, in some parts of the country a twelve week course is on offer. This consists of:

● twelve days in college

● 120 hours on-ward experience

● a 2,500 word essay

- presentation of work.

You must be successful in both the written and practical work to pass the course. When you have successfully completed the study days and the ward experience, you may return to practice. Your essay and practical ward experience may gain you 20 credits, out of the 120 required, towards a diploma in nursing.

Funding the 12 week course

Prior to 1999 you had to pay for these courses. In 1998 a twelve week course would have cost you £780. The government is encouraging qualified nurses back in to the profession and as a result 'back to nursing' courses are free for the forseeable future.

BEING SUPERVISED

If, even after your refresher course, you still lack confidence, don't worry. You will not be expected to work without help. For about six months after you return to work – or longer if you are working part-time – you will be under the supervision of a nurse mentor. He or she will be an experienced nurse who has practised in your particular work area for some time.

At first you may find that nothing is as you remembered it. New technology has changed some of the techniques to make nursing safer and easier for both nurses and patients. You may also find you are performing duties once done by a doctor:

- giving intravenous drugs

- putting up intravenous infusions

- inserting urine catheters

- taking blood.

At first you may find all this bewildering. But don't worry. Each day you will gain more confidence as you realise that patients don't change. They still need the care you provide and your experience outside nursing – perhaps of bringing up a family or caring for an elderly relative – will enhance your practice.

You may have had first hand experience of worrying about your sick child or your elderly parents so you will be able to empathise more closely with the relatives of your patients.

JUGGLING FAMILY LIFE

As well as the worry of returning to work after a break, you will have the anxiety of making sure your family does not suffer as a result. You may find it difficult to work certain shifts but your employers will probably be able to work out suitable flexible working hours for you. You might be able to start work after 9.00 so you can take the children to school in the morning and then finish your shift in time to pick them up in the afternoon. Find out the possibilities when you apply for the post.

There are increased opportunities to work part-time. Teaching or practice nursing are two posts which may allow you more time with your family. Job sharing has also become popular recently. With a job-sharing partner you would be able to work out the hours which best suit each of you.

Juggling family life, household chores and a career will not be easy but polish up your organisational skills and overcome your lack of confidence and you will succeed.

Looking after the children

If you have small children, you may be able to take them to work with you during the school holidays. Many hospitals run inexpensive crèches so if you have small children, you can easily be contacted if there is a problem. There are also play schemes available during this period. These provide entertainment and care for your children while you are at work so you do not have to worry about them. If your hospital does not have a holiday play scheme, find out if there is one in your area. Write to Kids Club Network, 279–281 Whitechapel Road, London E1 1BY or phone them on (0171) 247 3009. They should be able to tell you the nearest play scheme in your area.

If your children are very small and you have no family nearby to look after them while you are at work, the organisation Gingerbread may be able to help you. The charges for their nurseries are reasonable and they also offer advice and support if you are a single parent. Their address is 33 Wellington Street, London WC2E 7NE.

CHECKLIST

● Find out about Return to Practice Programmes.

● Accept advice from your 'mentor'.

● Organise your family life.

CASE STUDY

Returning to work on a children's ward

Alison trained on the Project 2000 course and thoroughly enjoyed her work on a variety of wards. She worked for five years before giving up after she married and became pregnant. She had two little boys and, when the youngest started school, Alison felt she would like to return to nursing. She took a Return to Practice Programme for two weeks at St Bartholomew's College of Midwifery and Nursing and then returned to Barts where she had worked previously. She started work on the children's ward and found her experience as a mother invaluable in dealing with her small patients.

Her nurse mentor, Jo, was very helpful and her colleagues supportive. She worked part-time so she was able to be with her children when they were not at school. Her husband, Bruce, worked from home so sometimes he looked after the children if Alison had to work when they were not at school.

Alison says, 'I was very nervous when I first started work again – even after the course. Everything seemed so different and I was sure I'd never remember everything I was told. Even the silly little things bothered me at first – like finding certain solutions were now in sachets rather than bottles! But the patients were the same and needed all the care I could give them. Bringing up two small children and worrying about their ailments helped me to understand what the parents of my patients must be feeling. My colleagues have been wonderful. I couldn't have got through the first few weeks without them but I feel much more confident now.'

11

Looking at Careers related to Nursing

TRAINING TO BE A DENTAL NURSE

If you wish to take the National Certificate for Dental Nurses Examination, there are no formal entry requirements. To find out details contact the National Examining Board for Dental Nurses, 110 London Street, Fleetwood, Lancashire FY7 6EU.

The majority of dentists usually train their own dental nurses so no previous experience is necessary. However, they normally require a good general education with several GCSEs, possibly including English and Biology. If you train in this way, you are advised to study for the National Certificate for Dental Nurses on a part-time basis. Check for details at your local college of further education.

You may choose to take a full-time course in dental nursing. In this case, you should have two to four GCSEs preferably including English and Biology. The minimum age for entry is usually 16-17 but it varies between dental schools so you should check this. There is no upper age limit. The course lasts for one to two years and can be taken at various dental schools and hospitals.

Taking the course

On the course, theory will be combined with practical work. You will listen to lectures, have individual tuition and take part in small group seminars. A wide variety of subjects will be studied, including:

- anatomy and physiology

- use of dental materials and instruments

- sterilisation and prevention of cross-infection

- use of drugs

- anaesthesia

- orthodontics (the correction of irregularities in the jaws and teeth)

- oral surgery

- causes of decay

- gum disease

- preparation of fillings

- keeping dental records

- dental radiography

- dental health

- care of patients.

For the final examination you will have a written paper, an oral examination and some practical tests.

Working in various environments
As a trained dental nurse, you may have the opportunity to work in any of the following:

- dental surgery

- community health clinic

- dental hospital

- general hospital.

You may work with a single dentist in a small practice or be part of a large team of dentists and nurses.

Using your skills
To be a successful dental nurse, you must like people and have a friendly personality. In spite of modern technology, many people still dread a visit to the dentist so you must learn to show sympathy and understanding to the patients. Your verbal and written communication skills should be finely honed; brush up on your administration as you will have to keep detailed, accurate records. You must be well organised.

A sense of humour would be useful and you should be fit and healthy; you will have to stand for long periods of time without wilting!

Coping with the work
You provide valuable help to the dentist. In a small practice you may act as a receptionist as well as a nurse but in all practices you will certainly be responsible for making sure the patients' records are kept up to date.

All in the day's work

- Prepare the surgery for the day's work.

- Check and sterilise the instruments.

- Help the patients to relax and comfort them if necessary.

- Note down any details given by the dentist.

- Mix fillings.

- Prepare materials for impressions.

- Hold suction instrument in patient's mouth to remove saliva.

- Process and mount X-ray films.

- Clean up surgery at the end of the day.

- Check patient's records and send out reminders to those who need to make appointments.

Pay and conditions

Guidelines for minimum salaries for dental nurses have been agreed by the British Dental Association and the British Association of Dental Nurses:

- unqualified dental nurse: £4,992 – £8,704

- registered dental nurse: £7,772 – £9,904

However, these are only recommendations and you may find your employer does not choose to follow them.

If you work in a hospital, your salary may be agreed by the Whitley Council. In this case, as an 18 year old trainee, you could expect to earn about £6,693. After you've completed your training, your salary would be £9,064 rising to £11,369.

After three years' experience, you could then become a senior dental nurse with a correspondingly higher salary which could rise to over £14,000.

What about promotion?

For promotion purposes, it might be useful to acquire other qualifications:

- certificate in oral health education

- certificate in dental radiography

- certificate in conscious sedation

- teacher's certificate in further and adult education

- dental hygienist diploma

- dental therapy diploma.

For further information write to the British Association of Dental Nurses, 110 London Street, Fleetwood, Lancashire FY7 6EU.

Revising the points

- You can study for the National Certificate for Dental Nurses.

- Many dentists train their own nurses.

- Your work is varied.

- You must have good communication and organisational skills.

- You must be fit.

WORKING AS AN OCCUPATIONAL THERAPIST

Occupational therapy is a fast growing profession. As an occupational therapist, you would be doing a very valuable job aiding individuals to learn or re-learn skills which enable them to do more for themselves. You would be involved in the assessment and rehabilitation of individuals of all ages with a variety of physical and mental health problems. Your aim would be to help your patients to reach their maximum level of physical, social and recreational independence through specifically selected and graded activities. You will support your patients by building up their stamina and confidence and, if relevant, helping them to return to work.

Training as an occupational therapist

You must be over 18 and under 40 to train as an occupational therapist. The college entry requirement is five GCSEs (two of which must be at A level), the BTEC National Diploma or appropriate NVQs. You should have studied at least one science subject and A level Biology would be useful. If you are older and have been working as an OT aid, these requirements may be waived.

The degree course lasts for three years. If you already have a relevant first degree, you may do an accelerated course over two years. At least a third of the degree is fieldwork based; this is spread over the three years and you will gain clinical experience in various care settings. During the first year you will be given two placements, each of five weeks. Your practical experience during both of the following two years will be of ten weeks' duration. These sessions will enable you to observe, participate in and practice occupational therapy under supervision.

The rest of the course will consist of modules in various subject areas. You will have lectures, tutorials, seminar discussions and workshops. There will be continuous assessment as well as examinations. All the modules must be passed before you can go on to the following year.

The third year contains a research element and a dissertation is required; in this you must illustrate your knowledge and practical experience of a particular aspect of occupational therapy.

Finding a post

When you have obtained your degree, you must register with the Council for Professions Supplementary to Medicine (CPSM) in order to practise with the NHS. There is a great demand for occupational therapists so you should have no difficulty in finding a suitable post.

The rates of pay are comparable with those of registered nurses. To find out more about training and working as an OT contact the College of Occupational Therapists, 106–114 Borough High Street, London SE1 1LB. Tel: (0171) 357 6480.

Experiencing a variety of settings

It is advisable that your first post should be a rotational one; you would then have the opportunity to see different aspects of the work. You might then choose to specialise in either the physical or the psychological areas. You might work in any of the following:

- a hospital

- a rehabilitation centre

- a day centre

- a health centre

- a residential home

- a nursery

- a unit catering for those with learning disabilities

- a mainstream school

- a special school

- a college.

You may work with very small children or the elderly; you may help disabled people of any age. You will have the opportunity to visit the patient's home to see what adaptations are needed to enable him or her to live more independently.

If you are working in a hospital, you will work as a team with other health care professionals; later you will help the patient to adjust after being discharged from hospital. You will often work closely with voluntary organisations.

Assessing your patients

You will be involved in standardised assessments and functional assessments. You may have to assess the individual in the home environment. The two key acronyms are PADL (Personal Activities of Daily Living) and DADL (Domestic Activities of Daily Living).

Examples

PADL	DADL
Dressing	Making a pot of tea
Washing	Dusting
Brushing hair	Making a bed

Your assessment notes would be filed and also passed on to social services, the patient's GP and any other involved professionals.

Specialities in occupational therapy

Physical rehabilitation	– head injury
	– orthopaedics
	– terminal and palliative care
	– HIV and AIDS
	– stroke patients
	– elderly patients
	– surgery
	– young disabled patients
Learning disability	
Mental health services	– child, family and carer situations
	– drug and alcohol abuse
	– elderly patients
	– forensic psychiatry and prison work

Paediatrics

Primary care

Environmental adaptations

Health promotion

Seeking promotion

With a variety of experience behind you, you could specialise in your chosen area. A variety of courses is offered. You might then choose to go into research, teaching or management. You might enjoy working as a 'care manager'. This job involves designing 'care packages'. You would work closely with housing agencies designing appropriate adaptations and modifications to houses which would enable disabled inhabitants to live independently.

Revising the points

● The three year course leads to an honours degree in occupational therapy.

● A third of the course is practical.

● Ideally your first post should be rotational to give you a variety of experience.

● There is a variety of areas in which you could specialise.

BEING A PHYSIOTHERAPIST

A physiotherapist concentrates on helping people through natural therapies. These include exercise, massage, manipulation and heat, light and electric treatment. The work is diverse and offers a great deal of opportunity.

Training to be a physiotherapist

To become a qualified physiotherapist and a member of the Chartered Society of Physiotherapists, you must complete a three or four year degree course. The entry requirements vary between universities but the usual ones are A levels, one of which should be a biological science and five GCSEs including maths, English and a science. If a BTEC national diploma in Health Studies or an advanced GNVQ in Health of Social Care or Science have been completed, these will be considered when you apply.

In addition to academic qualifications, the university will be looking for the following attributes in potential students:

- reliability and honesty

- good communication and caring skills

- ability to work independently

- sensitivity and tolerance

- enthusiasm, dedication and determination.

Applications from mature students are encouraged. Evidence of recent study including a foundation course in a science is required. To gain an insight into the work of a physiotherapist, it is necessary to work with one. You could work as an aid to a physiotherapist or as a voluntary worker in a physiotherapy department. If you have done so, this will be taken into account when you apply for training.

You will be university based for your first year but subsequent years include placements in various hospital departments and the community. To discover which universities are offering training and the entry requirements contact the Chartered Society of Physiotherapists at 14 Bedford Row, London WC1R 4ED. Tel: (0171) 306 6666.

Practising as a physiotherapist

As a physiotherapist, you will treat all age groups, offering them advice and educating them. You could work in any of the following departments:

- outpatients' clinic

- intensive care unit

- maternity department

- elderly wards

- stroke unit

- orthopaedics

- surgery unit.

Outside the hospital many more work opportunities exist. You may choose to work in industry, a hospice, the private sector or for a voluntary organisation. Your patients will require help in the following areas:

- arthritis

- replacement limbs

- mental illness

- at risk at work

- physical handicaps

- sports injuries

- paralysed limbs

- AIDS.

Teaching your patients

Much of your work will involve teaching patients to help themselves. In the field of mental illness, relaxation and fitness techniques are taught. In the maternity field, you will be involved with providing parentcraft classes where you will teach pre and post-natal exercises, birthing positions, breathing exercises and pelvic floor exercises.

You may also train others who are caring for the sick. You may teach nurses and carers how to lift safely and correctly. You may run rehabilitation classes for those recently suffering from a stroke or heart condition. You may have the opportunity to work with organisations which offer help to the disabled. You could be involved in a wide variety of work.

Revising the points

- You will study for a degree.

- Communication skills and a caring nature are essential.

- You will meet the old, young, well and sick.

- There is a wide variety of possible placements.

GOING INTO SOCIAL WORK

If you choose to go into social work, you will find that the problems you try to resolve and the people you meet will provide you with a varied and challenging job.

Training to be a social worker

The Diploma in Social Work (Dip. SW) is the professional qualification required to enable you to practise as a social worker. It is usually a full-time two year course although some universities offer part time courses. You should be at least 20 years old when starting the training. Entry requirements are three GCSEs and two A levels or an advanced GNVQ or a recognised access course.

Learning to practise
The methods used for learning are varied. Individual self-directed learning is encouraged but formal lectures, seminars, project work, presentations and role play are also used. You are likely to be given real life scenarios to resolve and you and your colleagues will be encouraged to criticise each other through video and role play.

Areas of study

● Human development.

● Social relationships.

● Legal studies.

● Sociology.

● Psychology.

● Social science.

During each year you will have a practical placement and will be supervised by a social worker who has completed a teaching course. You will be continuously assessed during your course on written assignments, examinations, presentations and practical work.

Working as a social worker

As a social worker, you will work as a team or alone in a variety of settings:

● hospitals

● social services departments

● children's homes

● residential care homes.

The nature of the work will vary depending on your setting. In a hospital you will work with occupational therapists, physiotherapists, nurses and doctors to assess the needs of a patient being discharged.

As a psychiatric social worker, you are usually based in a social services department. You would work as part of the community mental health care team beside psychiatric community nurses and doctors. Your role would be to support clients recovering from mental health problems. You may be required to take further training in this field.

If you work as part of a child and family care team, you will work closely with children's charities like the NSPCC and Dr Barnardo's. Wherever you choose to work no two days will be the same.

Further training

If you wish to continue your professional development or go into management or teaching, further training is required. There are 21 departments throughout the country which offer courses which have been approved by the Central Council for Education and Training in Social Work. Some are university based, while others expect you to provide evidence of learning while working as a social worker. For each programme, credit points are awarded and these can count towards a degree.

Recognised courses for social workers

● Child development and communication.

● Foundation in child protection.

● MA in social work.

● MSc in mental health social work.

● Diploma in family therapy.

● Positive parenting.

● Moving on with learning difficulties.

● Advanced social work studies in criminal justice.

● Social services management.

● Protection of vulnerable people.

● BSc (Hons) in health and community studies.

Revising the points

● To practise, a diploma in social work is required.

- You are likely to work as part of a team.

- You will work with children, families, the elderly or the mentally ill.

- A number of further training courses is available.

- Being a social worker can be a challenging job.

BECOMING A CHIROPODIST/PODIATRIST

Chiropodists, also known as podiatrists, will always be in demand as over 80 per cent of the population develop foot problems at some time during their lives. Older people, particularly, need regular foot care and with both men and women living longer than in the past, chiropodists are almost guaranteed permanent employment.

Training as a chiropodist

The minimum entry requirement to a degree course in chiropody is five GCSEs and two or three A levels. English should be one of your GCSE subjects and two science subjects are advisable. BTEC and GNVQ qualifications may also be accepted. You are advised to check with the appropriate university for its particular entry requirements. You may find some require higher qualifications than others. Mature students are usually accepted if they have taken an appropriate access course.

The degree course

Most degree courses last for three years full-time although some institutions offer part-time courses. Practical work will be combined with theory. During the first year half the course is likely to be practical. There will be an introductory life sciences course including anatomy and physiology. This will be followed by the study of theoretical chiropody and the principles of medicine and surgery relating to foot disorders. Other subjects you are likely to study will be:

- orthopaedics   –   foot deformities

- bacteriology   –   infection and how it spreads

- pedology   –   detailed study of healthy, diseased and deformed feet

- pharmacology –   the action of various drugs

- osteopathy   –   massage of the feet

- aetiology — study of the cause of disease
- pathology — study of the changes occurring in disease and deformity
- biomechanics — a mechanical science dealing with the movement of muscles and bones.

At the end of the course you will have both written and oral examinations. You will also have practical sessions where you may have to show and demonstrate appropriate appliances you have made.

Applying for state registration

State registration is essential if you wish to work for the NHS. You are eligible to apply for this once you have successfully completed a degree course which has been approved by the Council for Professions Supplementary to Medicine. Write to CPSN, Park House, 184 Kennington Park Road, London SE11 4BU. Tel: (0171) 582 0866.

If you choose to study at a privately funded centre, you may work privately but are not usually eligible for state registration. One of the oldest of the private institutions is the SMAE Institute (The Open College of Chiropody and Podiatry). Established in 1919, it is professionally recognised and is highly regarded in the private sector. The address is The New Hall, Bath Road, Maidenhead, Berkshire SL6 4LA. Tel: (01628) 621100.

Working as a chiropodist

As well as treating patients, you may work in an advisory capacity, giving talks in schools and health centres. Much of your practical work will be routine. You will deal with corns, warts, abrasions, blisters, toenail disorders, skin infections and other disorders. Many of your patients will be elderly so your treatment could be merely palliative. However, you can cure some conditions if you treat the problem early enough.

Treatment
You may use a variety of treatments to deal with different ailments:

- use of heat and cold
- exercises
- hydrotherapy (exercises in warm water)
- wax baths

- drugs and antiseptics

- dressings.

You may also have to perform minor operations on the foot or toenails under local anaesthetic.

Work environment
Most chiropodists who are state registered start work in the NHS and then move to private practice. You could work in a variety of settings:

- hospital

- clinic

- health centre

- school

- residential home

- private home.

Some industrial and commercial firms employ full or part time chiropodists and civilian chiropodists are employed by the Armed Services.

Pay and conditions
Full-time NHS chiropodists can earn from £12,635 to £19,880 and some senior posts command even higher salaries. Terms and conditions may vary from hospital to hospital and if you work in private practice, you can expect to earn considerably more.

If you work for the NHS, you will work about 37.5 hours for five days a week but in private practice your hours may be long and irregular. Part-time work is often available.

For further information contact the Society of Chiropodists and Podiatrists, 53 Welbeck Street, London W1M 7HE. Tel: (0171) 486 3381. The Institute of Chiropodists can be found at 27 Wright Street, Southport, Merseyside PR9 0TL. Tel: (01704) 546141.

Revising the points
- You will take a degree course.

- The work is varied.

- You can work in a variety of settings.

- You must be state registered to work in the NHS.

- If you train privately, you are not eligible for state registration.

WORKING FOR THE AMBULANCE SERVICE

The career structure of each ambulance service may vary as each is organised in regions but most shifts are from twelve hours so you would work from 7.00 to 19.00 or from 19.00 to 7.00. You are unlikely to work for more than five days in a row and will then have several days free.

Training as a care assistant

Most ambulance personnel start their training with a basic four week course which will qualify you as a care assistant. You would have a medical and an interview as well as being given a dictation and maths test. If you are successful, you will then start the four week course where you will study basic first aid and go out in an ambulance with an instructor.

When you have completed the course, you will do non-emergency work. You may be called upon to transfer patients from one hospital to another or ferry them to outpatients' departments or clinics. You will always work with a partner.

Training as a technician

After you have worked for six months to a year, you can apply to train as a technician. This is a more intensive course and lasts for six weeks. The entry examination lasts all day and is very gruelling. You would again be given a dictation and maths test and have to do a psychological profile where you tick appropriate answers to various questions. You would also have to have a fitness test which would probably include a 'back strength' test. If you fail this, you will not get on the course. Since it has been introduced, back injuries amongst ambulance crews have decreased considerably. Various practical tests will be included and you will go out in an ambulance with an instructor.

The course is divided into three sections with assessment throughout. For the first two weeks there is a detailed course including anatomy, physiology and related subjects; this is followed by a written exam. The second two weeks would be practical and you learn about everything that you are likely to meet on a job. You practise on dummy patients and take part in simulated accidents. The third part of the course consists of instruction in special procedures including advanced driving techniques.

While you are on the course, you will be paid and when you have completed it satisfactorily, you will be a trainee technician. At the end of a successful year's work during which you will be regularly assessed, you will be a fully qualified technician and awarded the National Ambulance Proficiency Certificate. Your pay will be increased. The salary for ambulance workers is reasonable and can always be increased by overtime.

Training as a paramedic

After a year's work as a qualified technician, you may apply for the paramedic course if your station officer will support you. It is likely that, in the future, this course may lead to a degree. It is divided into two sections, each of four weeks. During the first month you will study subjects in more depth and be given instruction in the use of drugs and how to give them as well as learning more practical skills.

During the second month you will work in a hospital where you will be assigned to a consultant who will assess you. You will gain experience of an operating theatre, an accident and emergency department and an intensive care ward.

The final exams and assessments are set by the NHS. Once you are fully qualified as a paramedic, you have to do two days' training every year to keep up to date and to polish up your skills.

Skills required by ambulance workers

- ability to work as a team

- common sense

- quick thinking

- able to work on your own initiative

- adaptability

- communication skills

- sense of humour

- patience

- concentration

- sympathy

- a calm attitude.

Being on call

Working for the ambulance service provides plenty of variety. It is a tiring but rewarding job. You will be called out for a variety of reasons – some serious, some minor and some even humorous. Beware of 999 calls dialled by small children who are playing with the phone! You will have to check the calls are genuine. You may have to deal with the following:

- asthma attack
- epilepsy
- heart attack
- accident in the home or in the workplace
- road traffic accident
- the aftermath of an explosion
- diabetic coma
- cot death
- drowning
- drug overdose.

You never know what the day may bring.

Revising the points

- Training to be a care assistant.
- Training to be a technician.
- Training to be a paramedic.

CASE STUDY

Rewarding times in the ambulance service

Richard worked for four years at various office jobs before deciding that he wanted to work for the ambulance service. He had four GCSEs and when he applied to be an ambulance care assistant, he was accepted.

He enjoyed the four week course and after qualifying, he spent a year on non emergency work, ferrying patients to hospital, taking them home after their discharge and transferring them from one hospital to another.

Then he applied for the more intensive six week technician course. He found it quite gruelling and was delighted to pass it. He was also relieved to pass the fitness test as several people he knew had failed it.

'The first time I was called to go out on an emergency, I was really nervous,' he said. 'Even now after three years I still jump when the phone goes.'

He enjoys the variety of work and the feeling of being of service to the public. With the rest of the ambulance crew, he has formed a good relationship with the police as they often have to work together.

'Sometimes, if we've had a 999 call and we can't get into the house, the police have to break down the door. A lot of our work is fairly basic but sometimes, of course, we have to attend horrific incidents. Some of the injuries I've seen have been terrible and we feel so helpless when we can't do anything to help. We have to try not to get emotionally involved but it's often quite hard especially if there is a child involved.'

Richard says that he finds the work very tiring and it tends to take over his life because of the twelve hour shifts. But he finds it very rewarding and has applied to take the paramedic course.

Glossary

Acupuncture. A treatment using needles inserted into the skin at specific points to relieve pain.

Anaesthetic. A drug which causes a loss of consciousness and/or sensation.

Aromatherapy. A treatment using essential oils through massage, inhalation, compresses and baths.

Audit. A systematic, critical analysis of the quality of care.

Caesarean section. The delivery of a baby through an incision in the abdomen.

Detoxification or detoxication. The process of neutralising or removing a poison in the body.

Diabetes. A disease involving the body's regulation of sugar.

Epilepsy. Fits due to electrical disorders in the brain.

Gastroenterology. The study of diseases of the bowel, stomach and intestines.

Gynaecology. The study of diseases of the female genital tract.

Herbalism. A treatment using medicinal herbs.

Homeopathy. A treatment of diseases using a small amount of a drug which causes symptoms of the disease in a healthy person.

Hypertension. High blood pressure.

Hypnosis. An artificially induced state of sleep.

Hypothermia. A seriously low body temperature.

Incontinent. Unable to control the loss of urine.

Intravenous. In a vein.

Obstetrics. The branch of medicine which deals with pregnancy, labour and the first six weeks of the post-natal period.

Orthopaedics. A field of surgery correcting problems with bones and joints.

Paediatrics. The branch of medicine dealing with children.

Palliative care. The relief of symptoms from an incurable disease.

Paramedic. A person associated with the medical profession.

Paranoia. A mental disorder where delusions of grandeur or persecution feature.

Phlebotomy. Taking blood from a vein.

Phobia. An irrational fear.

Pneumonia. Inflammation of the lung.

Primary nursing. A nursing method where a qualified nurse is responsible for a group of patients for the entire duration of their care.

Prostate. A gland found in males which is positioned near the bladder.

Psoriasis. A chronic skin condition.

Reflexology. A therapy where pressure is applied to specific zones on the feet to alleviate health problems.

Rehabilitation. A programme which aims to help a disabled or convalescing patient to a state of maximum physical capability.

Scan. A two dimensional picture of a part of the body by using a machine.

Shiatsu. A therapy where pressure is placed on specific parts of the body to prevent or relieve a problem or for relaxation.

Stoma care. Looking after an artificial opening on the body as a result of surgery.

Therapeutic touch. Touching a patient to help treat or relieve symptoms of a health problem.

Tuberculosis. An infectious disease where small swellings occur mainly in the lungs.

Urology. The branch of medicine which specialises in the urinary and genital systems.

Further Reading

REFERENCE BOOKS

Careers in Nursing and Related Professions, Linda Nazarko (Kogan Page, 7th edition).

Baillieres Nurses' Dictionary, Kesner and Tindall (Bailliere and Tindall).

Black's Medical Dictionary, edited by C W H Havard (A & C Black).

Blackwell's Dictionary of Nursing.

Career Development for Nurses – Opportunities and Options, Jane Sanderson (Scutari Press).

Developing your Career in Nursing, D. Cormack (Chapman and Hall).

Living and Working in Saudi Arabia, Rosalie Rayburn and Kate Bush (How To Books, 2nd edition).

Living and Working in America, Steve Mills (How To Books, 4th edition).

Living and Working in Australia, Laura Veltman (How To Books, 6th edition).

NURSING JOURNALS

British Journal of Community Nursing
British Journal of Health Care Management
British Journal of Learning Disabilities
British Journal of Midwifery
Cancer Nursing
Complementary Therapies in Nursing and Midwifery
Community Nurse
Community Practitioner
Elderly Care
Emergency Nurse
Health Service Journal
Health Trends
Journal of Advanced Nursing
Journal of Medical Ethics

Journal of Paediatrics
Mental Health Practice
Nurse Researcher
Nurse Education Today
Nursing Times
Nursing Management
Nursing Standard
Paediatric Nursing
Practice Nurse
Professional Nurse

Useful Addresses

Association of Nursery Training Colleges, The Princess Christian College, 26 Wilbraham Road, Fallowfield, Manchester M14 6JX.

Australian High Commission, Australia House, Strand, London WC2B 4LA.

Australian Nursing Council Inc, GPO Box 1907, Canberra, ACT 2601, Australia.

Boarding Schools Association, Ysgol Nant, Valley Road, Llanfairfechan, Gwynedd, North Wales LL33 0ES. Tel: (01248) 680542.

British Association for Counselling, 1 Regent Place, Rugby CV21 2PJ.

British Association of Dental Nurses, 110 London Street, Fleetwood, Lancashire FY7 6EU.

Chartered Society of Physiotherapists, 14 Bedford Row, London WC1R 4ED. Tel: (0171) 306 6666.

College of Occupational Therapists, 106–114 Borough High Street, London SE1 1LB. Tel: (0171) 357 6480.

Commission on Graduates of Foreign Nursing Schools (CGFNS), Fulbright House, 62 Doughty Street, London WC1N 2LS.

Contributions Agency, Class 2 Group, DSS, Newcastle-upon-Tyne NE98 1YX.

Council for Professions Supplementary to Medicine, Park House, 184 Kennington Park Road, London SE11 4BU. Tel: (0171) 582 0866.

Department of Trade and Industry, European Division, Ashdown House, 6th floor, 123 Victoria Street, London SW1E 6RB.

Employment Service, Deputy Chief Nursing and Healthcare Employment Consultant, Broadacre House, Market Street (East), Newcastle-upon-Tyne NE1 6HQ.

Employment Service, Overseas Placing Unit, Rockingham House, 123 West Street, Sheffield S1 4ER.

English National Board Careers Service, PO Box 2EN, London W1A 2EN. Tel: (0171) 391 6200 or (0171) 391 6205.

Gingerbread, 33 Wellington Street, London WC2E 7NE.

Institute of Chiropodists, 27 Wright Street, Southport, Merseyside PR9 0TL. Tel: (01704) 546141.

International Health Exchange, 8–10 Dryden Street, London WC2E 9NA.

Kids Club Network, 279–281 Whitechapel Road, London E1 1BY. Tel: (0171) 247 3009.

National Examining Board for Dental Nurses, 110 London Street, Fleetwood, Lancashire FY7 6EU.

National Nursery Examination Board, 8 Chequer Street, St Albans, Hertfordshire AL1 3XZ.

Nursing Adviser, HM Prison Service Health Care, Cleland House, Page Street, London SW1P 4LN.

Nursing and Midwifery Admissions Service (NMAS), Fulton House, Jessop Avenue, Cheltenham, Glos GL50 3SH.

Open College of Chiropody and Podiatry, The New Hall, Bath Road, Maidenhead, Berkshire SL6 4LA. Tel: (01628) 621100.

Royal College of Nursing, 20 Cavendish Square, London W1M 0AB.

Society of Chiropodists and Podiatrists, 53 Welbeck Street, London W1M 7HE. Tel: (0171) 486 3381.

Index

PASSING THAT INTERVIEW
Your step-by-step guide to coming out on top

Judith Johnstone

Using a systematic and practical approach, this book takes you step-by-step through the essential pre-interview groundwork, the interview encounter itself, and what you can learn from the experience. The book contains sample pre- and post-interview correspondence, and is complete with a guide to further reading, glossary of terms, and index. 'This is from the first class How To Books stable.' *Escape Committee Newsletter*. 'Offers a fresh approach to a well documented subject.' *Newscheck* (Careers Service Bulletin). 'A complete step-by-step guide.' *The Association of Business Executives*. Judith Johnstone is a Member of the Institute of Personnel & Development; she has been an instructor in Business Studies and adult literacy tutor, and has long experience of helping people at work.

144pp illus. 1 85703 538 0. 5th edition.

WRITING A CV THAT WORKS
Developing and using your key marketing tool

Paul McGee

What makes a CV stand out from the crowd? How can you present yourself in the most successful way? This practical book shows you how to develop different versions of your CV for every situation. Reveal your hidden skills, identify your achievements and learn how to communicate these successfully. Different styles and uses for a CV are examined, as you discover the true importance of your most powerful marketing tool. Paul McGee is a freelance Trainer and Consultant for one of Britain's largest out-placement organisations. He conducts marketing workshops for people from all walks of life.

128pp illus. 1 85703 365 5. 2nd edition.

GETTING THAT JOB
The complete job finders handbook

Joan Fletcher

Now in its fourth edition this popular book provides a clear step-by-step guide to identifying job opportunities, writing successful application letters, preparing for interviews and being selected. 'A valuable book.' *Teachers Weekly*. 'Cheerful and appropriate . . . particularly helpful in providing checklists designed to bring system to searching for a job. This relaxed, friendly and very helpful little book could bring lasting benefit.' *Times Educational Supplement*. 'Clear and concise . . . should be mandatory reading by all trainees.' *Comlon Magazine* (LCCI). Joan Fletcher is an experienced Manager and Student Counsellor.

112pp illus. 1 85703 380 9. 4th edition.

IMPROVING YOUR WRITTEN ENGLISH
How to sharpen up your grammar, punctuation and spelling for everyday use

Marion Field

This user-friendly book will be a boon for anyone who needs to brush up his or her English. Written in short, easily understandable sections, it deals with the basics of writing good English. There are sections on punctuation, sentence construction, and spelling. All the common pitfalls are tackled: when to use apostrophes and how to spell those frequently misspelt words. The reader is shown how to adopt the different styles needed for writing a report, essay or short story. Useful exercises and illustrations are included throughout the book. Marion Field has taught English in a variety of secondary schools. For many years she was Head of English in a large Comprehensive School and she is also an examiner for GCSE English.

128pp illus. 1 85703 358 2. 2nd edition.